PERSONALITY DISORDERS IN CHILDREN AND ADOLESCENTS

PERSONALITY DISORDERS IN CHILDREN AND ADOLESCENTS

PAULINA F. KERNBERG, M.D.
ALAN S. WEINER, PH.D.
KAREN K. BARDENSTEIN, PH.D.

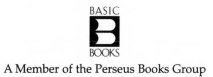

BASIC BOOKS

A Member of the Perseus Books Group

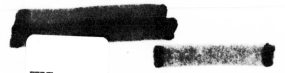

Library of Congress Cataloging-in-Publication Data
Kernberg, Paulina F.
    Personality disorders in children and adolescents / Paulina F. Kernberg,
Alan S. Weiner, Karen K. Bardenstein.
        p. cm.
    Includes bibliographical references and index.
    ISBN 0-465-09562-3
    1. Personality disorders in children.   2. Personality disorders in adolescence.
3. Child psychiatry.   I. Weiner, Alan S.   II. Bardenstein, Karen K.   III. Title.
[DNLM: 1. Personality Disorders—Adolescence.   2. Personality Disorders—
Child. WS 350.8.P3 K39p 1999]
RJ506.P32 K47 1999
618.92'89—dc21   99–046470
                                                                                       CIP

00   01   02   03   /   10   9   8   7   6   5   4   3   2   1

To my father,
Isaac S. Fischer

Contents

PART IV:
THE BORDERLINE PERSONALITY ORGANIZATION

PART V:
THE PSYCHOTIC PERSONALITY ORGANIZATION

PART VI:
SPECIAL ISSUES AND RESEARCH IMPLICATIONS

Preface

Personality disorders (PDs) in adulthood have been recognized as having a profound and prolonged impact on the individual, on the family, and on society (Ruegg and Frances 1995). Epidemiological research indicates a high prevalence of PDs between the ages of 9 and 19 as well (Bernstein et al. 1993); however, the development of PDs in young people has not received the attention it merits.

Our purpose is to present the mounting and compelling evidence for the presence of PDs in children and adolescents so that they will be more readily recognized and treated. In this population, they are associated with increased suicidality, delinquency, academic failure, social dysfunction, and substance abuse. They also worsen the prognosis for patients suffering from such other disturbances as anxiety disorders, affective disorders, and eating disorders.

All clinical and research findings about adult PDs emphasize their early developmental precursors. Yet the very existence of PDs in children and adolescents has been questioned. Practically, PDs often require more extended and therefore more costly treatment than that covered by third-party payers. Conceptually, there persists an understandable reluctance to believe that a developing child can have a disorder of such magnitude that it interferes with his relationship to his environment and to himself.

Because of the ongoing debate (P. Kernberg 1990, Shapiro 1990), we think it is timely to focus more systematically on this issue. It is our intention to highlight the usefulness of a developmental perspective for identifying the features of PDs and related pathological personality traits at different developmental phases. We will provide clinical and research evidence to support the reliable identification of PDs in children and adolescents.

The first section begins by introducing the developmental perspective on personality and personality disorders: It reports epidemiological findings and examines the *DSM* nosology, including its influence on research and clinical practice as it applies to PDs in children and adolescents. There follows a discussion of basic components of personality, such as temperament, identity, gender, and defense mechanisms. Then, we review methods of assessing a child's patterns of behavior and the mental status findings that reflect personality traits—historical information, structured and unstructured interviews, psychological testing, and biological techniques.

The second section covers the various types of PDs, subgrouped according to level of personality organization and ranging from lesser to greater severity, from neurotic through borderline to psychotic personality organization.

The final section opens by addressing special issues concerning the relationship of PDs to questions of gender identity, suicidality, and substance abuse and to such social factors as cultural background and divorce. It moves on to problems of nomenclature of the childhood and adolescent syndromes in *DSM-IV* and concludes with an overview of directions for research.

The differences in length among the various chapters correlate with the differential experience of the authors in dealing with the different categories of PDs and also with the variable state of the field as we surveyed it. We hope that having a framework in common with adult PDs will facilitate longitudinal research in the childhood and adolescent arenas and that new data and new categories will be added as the results of such research and also clinical evidence accumulate. Meanwhile, there will be a footprint, like the Periodic Table of Elements.

We want to acknowledge with thanks our colleagues who supported our efforts and also those colleagues who questioned the whole idea. John Newman saw the beginnings of the work and organized the initial manuscripts. Thanks go to him, and to Raquel Reid-McFarlane, who took on the arduous task of transcribing the first versions. Special thanks go to Lois Macri, who weaved in and out of the thicket of versions of chapters and negotiated the web of communications with authors and editors. A garland of thanks goes to Nina Gunzenhauser, who made us better—much better—with her editorial comments, and to Cindy Hyden for her unwavering support and for leading us to the end of the voyage.

We three authors hope this book stimulates others to pursue research based on the concepts developed within it, as well as clinical training and practice in the field.

Paulina F. Kernberg
Alan S. Weiner
Karen K. Bardenstein

PART I
DEVELOPMENTAL PERSPECTIVE

CHANGING VIEWS OF PERSONALITY DISORDERS

Whereas clinicians and academicians have long taken an interest in personality and its variations, they have understandably focused more on Axis I disorders than on personality disorders. One reason may be that the impact of PDs may be less readily apparent. Chronic schizophrenia and major affective disorders are defined by signs and behaviors that are readily observed, described, and measured: It is easier to inquire about a hallucination than to inquire about patterns of behavior that indicate the presence of an identity disturbance.

Because personality disorders involve more extensive aspects of individual functioning, reaching a consensus on criteria for their incidence is more complicated. For example, two longitudinal projects that examined community samples and used respected but different measurement tools with different criteria provided quite different pictures of the prevalence of PDs in adolescence. The Bernstein et al. study (1993) cited earlier used a variety of measures to arrive at its rates (31.2/moderate and 17.2/severe), whereas the other study (Lewinsohn et al. 1997) used the personality disorder examination, a structured interview format developed for adults (Loranger 1988) and found that 3.3 percent of their young adult subjects had a PD.

Moreover, research on Axis I disorders has provided a window for studying the brain and its functioning, leading to the development of pharmacological interventions that have continued to evolve and to progress. By contrast, the role of pharmacological intervention for PDs is less clear, as are the potential brain-behavior relationships. Even though the treatment of those PD features associated with Axis I problems (e.g., mood) can be approached pharmacologically and can be relatively brief, the interpersonal features of a PD often necessitate intensive psychotherapy, which is less likely to be supported by third-party payers, who emphasize less expensive, less inclusive, and briefer treatment.

Despite these difficulties, the study of PDs in adults has been drawing steadily increasing interest: A journal devoted specifically to PDs was founded in 1987 (*The Journal of Personality Disorders*), and PD research now appears regularly in diverse psychiatry and psychology journals. Changes in the representation of PDs in *The Diagnostic and Statistical Manual of Mental Disorders* have certainly been influential (Livesley 1995). The third edition (*DSM-III* 1980) created diagnostic criteria for each PD and introduced the multiaxial system that distinguished personality disorders (Axis II) from all other mental disorders (Axis I). This system of classification, further refined by continued reliability and validity studies in *DSM-III-Revised* (1987) and *DSM-IV* (1994), has allowed for the independent examination of a patient for the presence of one or more PDs and has facilitated identification of the co-occurrence of personality disorders with other disorders.

DSM-IV defines *personality traits* as "enduring patterns of perceiving, relating to, and thinking about the environment and oneself that are exhibited in a wide range of social and personal contexts" (p. 630). A *personality disorder*, in turn, is defined as

> an enduring pattern of inner experience and behavior that deviates markedly from the expectations of the individual's culture, is pervasive and inflexible, has an onset in adolescence or early adulthood, is stable over time (and across a broad range of personal and social situations), and leads to distress or impairment (p. 630).

Thus, in line with research and clinical findings, a PD is expected to have a serious impact on most spheres of a person's life, including behavior at work or at school, interaction with peers and family, and cognitive and emotional functioning reflecting his sense of self and others and his relationship with reality in general. This formulation requires a complex and comprehensive approach to assessment and integration of information.

THE CONCEPT OF PERSONALITY DISORDER IN CHILDREN AND ADOLESCENTS

Although changes in the *DSM* system encouraged clinical interest and research on PDs in adulthood, it has not had a similar impact on the study of the onset and course of PDs in children and adolescents. For reasons both personal and theoretical, clinicians have been reluctant to make the diagnosis of a personality disorder in children and adolescents.

One reason for this reluctance is that all professionals who deal with children have reservations about labeling them with a diagnosis that implies severity and nonmalleability. There is concern that a PD label, like that of other serious psychological disorders, will adversely affect the child's (or her family's) self-concept or prejudice her future by appearing somewhere in her personal record. However, failing to diagnose a PD in the child could also jeopardize her future by making it difficult or impossible for her to obtain necessary and appropriate treatment. Ironically, on the basis of the prevailing *DSM-IV* definition, insurance companies in the era of managed care are not always willing to recognize that children have PDs, and the clinician who makes the diagnosis may be told that it is not "listed in our computer for patients of that age." Accordingly, treatment for a PD diagnosis may not be supported by third-party payers; in general, a personality disorder is not a candidate for a managed care approach.

Some scientists and clinicians believe that personality has not yet crystallized in children or adolescents; for them, the very existence of a personality disorder would not make sense. Others (see, for example, Shapiro 1990) question only whether a PD can be diagnosed before adolescence, when an adult-like identity is thought to coalesce (Blos 1967, Erikson 1968). This approach is basically nondevelopmental because it does not consider the process by which, at each phase of development, an age-appropriate identity and personality are formed. Ignoring the developmental line of the structuring of identity means ignoring the ways in which personality development can be adversely affected at any age.

PERSONALITY DISORDERS AND DEVELOPMENT

The *DSM-IV* definition has clear developmental implications although it fails to address them. The system appears to be struggling with issues related to the first emergence or appearance of a behavior or trait; its relationship, if any, to the final (that is, adult) form; and whether or not the behavior or trait demonstrates stability over time and/or continuity with behaviors or traits seen later in development. These are issues about which scientists interested in the developmental process have long been concerned.

The Emergence of Personality Traits in Childhood

Research during the past several decades has uncovered considerable knowledge about the child's developing personality, including emergence of a sense of identity, affect modulation, thinking style, and relationship with the external world, that has implications for the development of PDs in children. With respect to the development of a sense of self, for example, it has been found that recognition of oneself by name in a mirror occurs by 3 years of age; a sense of shame, implying self-consciousness, emerges before 2 years of age (Lewis 1993). Another example, impulsivity, which has a bio-logical-temperamental basis and, when maladaptive, is an intrinsic compo-nent of a borderline personality disorder (*DSM-IV*), is seen early in development and becomes modulated with age (Achenbach et al. 1995, Bernstein et al. 1993). Empathy is yet another example: A basic component of interpersonal functioning because of its role in the relationship between self and others, empathy develops in early childhood (Hoffman 1977), evidenc-ing clear signs by 2 years of age. Deviations in empathy are a component of some PDs, particularly narcissistic and antisocial disorders (Selzer et al. 1987).

Another component of personality—thinking style and the presence of a concrete operational reasoning system (Piaget 1950)—is apparent by middle childhood and persists into adulthood. Differences in style of language ex-pression have been distinguished among school-age children, such as the distinction between "sharpeners," whose style is analytic and detailed, and "levelers," whose expression is global and affect-laden (Gardner and Mori-arty 1968). A thought disorder can also be reliably identified through an in-terview and is diagnostically significant by this age (Caplan 1994).

Reality testing, thought processes, and disordered thinking can be reliably measured in school-age children with the Rorschach technique (Exner and Weiner 1995). These Rorschach measures show stability across time and are valid predictors of impairment in basic components of personality function-ing. For example, one study (Roseby et al. 1995) reported on Rorschach find-ings in children aged 9 to 13 years in high-conflict divorce situations. Years after the divorce, almost 100 percent of the children who had experienced high-conflict divorce (versus 10 percent of control children) produced Rorschach responses indicative of heightened levels of distrust, low self-esteem, concreteness, constriction, hypervigilance, and alienation from oth-ers, with excessive self-reliance.

STABILITY AND DEVELOPMENT OF PERSONALITY TRAITS

Both the stability of psychological characteristics and the possibility of or-dered, systematic change across developmental periods have been studied for many years (see, for example, Achenbach et al. 1995, Bloom 1964, Brim and Kagan 1980, Kagan and Moss 1962). J. Kagan (1969) introduced the con-cept of heterotypic continuity to describe those situations in which there is a significant correlation between two seemingly dissimilar variables mea-sured at two widely different points in time—for example, imperviousness to reward and punishment in early childhood with lack of remorse and empathy in the antisocial personality. When such a correlation occurs, the investigator introduces some theoretical explanation to account for the association because the assumption is that there must be some connection between the variables.

The concept of heterotypic continuity has been useful and important in longitudinal analyses of behaviors. It is not possible to measure the same variable in the same way at different points in development and find stability across periods because the expression and meaning of a behavior changes from one period to another. For example, intelligence, one component of personality, cannot be measured with the same test items at different developmental periods. Traditional infant intelligence tests do not predict later intellectual functioning (McCall 1979). However, when information processing and attention are measured in ways that are appropriate for each developmental level, a relationship can be seen between infant cognitive functioning and intelligence in late childhood (Slater 1995).

Attachment

The study of attachment is of fundamental importance for thinking about continuity across developmental periods because patterns of attachment continue to determine characteristics of interpersonal relations and the individual's mental representation of others. In our opinion, attachment classifications should also be viewed as descriptors of personality styles that influence the individual's patterns of interactions with others; it is this relationship that accounts for the continuity of attachment patterns with later functioning.

Strikingly, researchers have found a correspondence between the classification of subtypes of toddlers' attachment behaviors in the Strange Situation procedure (Ainsworth et al. 1978) and interview-derived adult attachment status. The Adult Attachment Interview (AAI) (Main and Goldwyn 1994) is used to assess the individual's internal representation of the attachment relation. In effect, both the Strange Situation and the AAI are designed to measure the attachment relation, which is thought to be a continuous feature of the personality that manifests itself in different ways over the course of development and appears to be transmitted transgenerationally (Benoit and Parker 1994).

The coherence of the attachment construct is supported by the findings of longitudinal studies performed by A. Sroufe and his colleagues (Sroufe

1997). Infants who show an avoidant attachment with their caregivers may not only show superficial relationships later in childhood but, because of their inability to take an empathic stance with others, may display aggression, bullying, and conduct disorders in later childhood. Infants who display a resistant attachment, rejecting comfort when it is offered, do not grow up to show an oppositional-defiant disorder as might be expected. Instead, they develop chronic vigilance, a personality trait, and show an increased likelihood of developing some form of anxiety disorder.

In another study (1993), Sroufe and his colleagues also reported impressive relationships between patterns of attachment assessed in the laboratory in the Strange Situation from 12 to 18 months of age and diverse social behaviors, such as peer interactions and self-reliance, in middle childhood and adolescence. Thus, Sroufe has been able to demonstrate heterotypic continuity across lengthy time periods by emphasizing the predictive significance of dyadic relationships in which the individual's construction of self and other elicits predictable reactions from others that reinforce and maintain behavior patterns and internal models.

This approach differs from one that attributes the apparent continuity of attachment-related behaviors to the stability of the environment in which the child is developing (Magai and Hunziker 1993). It postulates, rather, that the child constructs and codetermines his environment. Features in the child, such as temperament, can contribute to the formation and implementation of caretaking behaviors that are sadomasochistic or narcissistic.

Three Patterns of Interaction

A. Caspi (Caspi and Bern 1990, Caspi and Moffitt 1995) has described three patterns of person-environment interaction (which may have temperamental and genetic sources) that are useful for thinking about how personality traits work to sustain themselves and maintain continuity in functioning across time and situation. Personality traits themselves may be viewed as patterns of interactions that induce experiences and reactions from others.

In *evocative interactions*, the individual draws forth particular responses from others. For instance, impulsive, inattentive children elicit more punitive, coercive behaviors from adults than do easy-to-manage children. In personality formation, the masochistic individual, for example, also induces others to react in mutually reinforcing ways to maintain the trait.

In *reactive interactions*, different youngsters interpret and react differently to the same situation. K. Dodge and colleagues (1986) have described how aggressive elementary school–aged boys perceive neutral acts by others as having an aggressive, hostile intent. Anxious children, by contrast, are more likely to react to an event as if it had a fearful component.

In *proactive interactions*, the individual creates or seeks situations compatible with her personality or interactional style. Friendship patterns belong here. Caspi and Bern (1990) suggest that proactive interactions increase with age and autonomy and may account for the positive change, with age, in the stability of correlations across time.

STABILITY AND PSYCHOPATHOLOGY IN CHILDHOOD

A general assumption often made by practitioners is that children are changeable and malleable and that the developmental process propels the child toward change, if not toward a healthy outcome itself, in which many psychological and behavioral problems can be outgrown. Nevertheless, there are children who fulfill the *DSM-IV* criteria for a PD in which the maladaptive personality traits appear to be pervasive and persistent. Yet *DSM-IV* traces the onset of a PD only to adolescence and early adulthood, not to early childhood.

Although many problems at the preschool level resolve themselves, it is not true that all children's problems are transitory, especially in school-aged children. Given the complexity of development, it is remarkable that there is any predictability of adult psychopathology from early childhood (Kagan 1997). Many examples from a variety of domains of functioning indicate a continuity in problem behavior.

Kagan and Zentner (1996) reviewed longitudinal studies to examine the possible relationship between adult psychopathology and childhood problems that occur before 4 years of age. They concluded that in preschool children extreme impulsivity may be a forerunner of adolescent antisocial behavior and that shyness may be a precursor of an avoidant personality. Kagan and Zentner suggest that the factors contributing to a relation between early childhood problems and later Axis I and Axis II disorders include temperament, an environment that enhances the temperament-based psychological vulnerabilities, and stressors that generate symptoms.

Our clinical experience indicates that most children who are seen at an outpatient clinic setting have had their disorder for more than two years. For instance, selective mutism—a relatively unusual symptom that may be a manifestation of a personality trait, shyness, and/or social anxiety—often is not diagnosed until the child is in kindergarten or 1st grade, yet it has an early age of onset. Parents report that the child has always displayed this quality (Dow et al. 1995), and Black and Uhde (1995) report that the selectively mute children they examined showed an average duration of the disorder of 5.7 years.

As another example, a clear, reliable distinction can be made between childhood-onset and adolescent-onset antisocial behavior. The childhood-onset variety of antisocial behavior has a long-term life course. It is associated with specific early temperamental and neuropsychological factors (e.g., impulsivity and language and memory, respectively), and it is related to the later development of antisocial personality disorders (Moffitt et al. 1996). We may assume that abnormal development continues through abnormal pathways and that children tend to maintain their psychological disturbances, especially when untreated, thereby meeting the criteria for persistence and pervasiveness of maladaptive traits.

P. Cohen and colleagues (Cohen et al. 1993) studied the persistence of childhood disorders and concluded from their epidemiological data that psychiatric disorders in childhood may be as stable as those in adulthood. Likewise, Costello and Angold (1995), in a review of developmental epidemiology, indicated that there is continuity to the child's vulnerability and that the presence of a childhood disorder significantly increases the likelihood of a disorder in adolescence. For example, in reviewing the Isle of Wight studies, they found a 46 percent prevalence rate for a psychiatric disorder in those adolescents who, as children, showed an emotional disorder and a 75 percent prevalence rate in adolescence for those who had shown a conduct disorder, compared with a 21 percent prevalence rate in adolescents who did not have a childhood psychiatric disorder. C. Kestenbaum (1983) reported that seven of the eight borderline children she carefully examined and followed did not show any remission. Another study (Lewinsohn et al. 1997) found that the presence of Axis I disorders earlier in childhood, especially more than two such diagnoses, greatly increases the likelihood of a personality disorder in later adolescence and young adulthood.

The hallmark of PDs is their inflexible, maladaptive qualities, and in our view it is these qualities of personality functioning that show continuity over time. Even though a particular behavior feature changes with development—and this should be expected—the maladaptive impact of the PD on the self and others persists. These maladaptive qualities are probably least evident when the child or adult finds himself in situations that are structured, nonchallenging, or predictable; they are more likely to appear in periods of change and stress.

Such periods can include activities that make greater interpersonal demands (for example, developing new friendships or establishing a level of intimacy in a relationship); that involve competition and risk of failure and humiliation (for example, taking a test, competing in team sports, or performing publicly at work); or that make new demands for autonomy (for example, agreeing to a sleep-over, beginning high school, or finding and performing at a job in the absence of authority or supervision).

In a clinical setting, one also sees that the clarity of the expression of a trait is influenced by the situation. For instance, in unstructured group situations antisocial individuals emerge as leaders because of their feelings of omnipotence. Nurses' reports on an inpatient unit, deriving from observations in less structured situations, can be more informative about personality traits than observations based on structured interviews (P. Kernberg et al. 1997).

In the absence of intervention from the environment, the manifestation of a PD would be expected to become more evident, intractable, and maladaptive with the new developmental demands associated with each developmental transition. Livson and Peskin (1967) reported that behaviors assessed in early adolescence (11 to 13 years of age) were better predictors of adult functioning than were similar behaviors assessed when the children were younger or in middle adolescence. Thus, how the child handles the transition between grade school and junior high school is a better predictor of how transitions will be handled later in life than are behaviors assessed during more stable periods in development. This finding may be explained by the characteristic defenses and coping mechanisms called upon in these situations as the youngster tries to deal with the anxieties brought on by developmental transitions.

However, what about situations that do not seem to show continuity? What is to be done if a child meets accepted diagnostic criteria for a PD at one stage, but this diagnosis does not show longitudinal stability to later developmental stages? Indeed, as we have noted, *DSM-IV* almost warns us to expect this situation. D. Bernstein and colleagues (Bernstein et al. 1996) report that PDs were not persistent in 43 percent of the adolescents they followed longitudinally. Does this mean that the initial diagnosis was wrong or that the child's functioning is still unstable, thereby indicating that the concept of a PD is not tenable in children?

It should be recognized that personality traits and personality disorders can and do change, not only in childhood and adolescence but also in adulthood. J. C. Perry (1993) reviewed longitudinal studies of adults diagnosed with a borderline personality disorder (BPD) and concluded that, after 10 years, 52 percent of the original patient group retained a "definite or probable" diagnosis of BPD, with 3.7 percent remitting every year. Furthermore, it is not unusual for adults to show comorbidity of personality disorder diagnoses from different Axis II clusters. There is also considerable heterogeneity within a personality disorder diagnosis; two individuals with a BPD diagnosis may manifest very different features of the disorder (Widiger and Trull 1992). Thus, a "pure type" is not readily identifiable, and adults should not serve as the gold standard for studying the stability of personality disorders in children. It would be unproductive to overlook this heterogeneity in adults but to use it to discredit the existence of PDs in children.

Our concern is that the *DSM-IV* standards may unwittingly discourage the diagnosis of PDs in children and may diminish the likelihood that clinicians and researchers will be willing to apply the diagnosis. Such a tendency would serve to confirm the *DSM* assumption but not provide the needed information for a proper evaluation of the position. In our view, there can be stability or coherence across time to many important aspects of the child's functioning that are relevant to how PDs are thought to develop.

At this time, we would endorse applying adult PD criteria to children. It is our belief that exemplars of these criteria can be identified in children in a reliable manner. Using this approach would provide an initial framework from which to proceed so that, over time, developmentally specific criteria can be identified that reflect developmental shifts and produce a more exact developmental psychopathology of personality and personality disorders.

Comparing personality-disordered children with non–personality-disordered children may prove to be more productive than comparing adults with children. The differences between infantile and pathological narcissism serve as an illustration: in the former, the young child wishes to be the center of attention and expects support while acknowledging dependency and expressing gratitude; the child with pathological narcissism also demands to be the center of attention but neither admits dependence nor expresses gratitude.

It is our perspective that PDs in children, like PDs in adults, are reliably identifiable, correlate with other Axis I and Axis II disorders, and show the pattern of persistence that makes their impact pervasive and severe.

I.2

Components of Personality

The study of personality focuses on individual differences. Although general experimental findings from biology, psychology, and psychiatry are indeed essential to that study, the particular goal is to discover and account for stable differences that characterize individuals or types of individuals and distinguish them from one another. One can then understand how such differences serve as modifiers of general human functioning.

This chapter describes salient variables in the development of children that contribute to the description, understanding, and treatment of personality disorders.

- *Temperament*—a biologically based disposition that influences the child's interaction with his world by affecting both the nature and style of the child's approach and the reactivity of others.
- *Identity*—an internal mental construction that involves the child's developing sense of self-sameness across time and situation.
- *Gender*—a fundamental dimension, itself a component of a developing identity, that defines individuals across cultures and embodies certain behavioral expectations; a dimension in which the type and frequency of psychopathology varies.
- *Neuropsychological Developmental Disorders*—deficits in cognitive and ego functioning that include neuropsychological processes and affect how the child may process, organize, and recall information.

- *Affect*—the child's emotional reactions and the internal, mental "glue" that links self- and other-representations.
- *Defense Mechanisms*—the child's characteristic mode of coping with and adapting to internal and external stress and, as such, an important element in the diagnosis and treatment of personality disorders.

These variable components of personality are, in part, influenced by the child's experiences, but they are also evocative factors that themselves influence the reactivity of the child's world and affect how the child interprets and constructs his experiences.

They are also fundamental to a definition of normal personality. A normal child or adolescent can be described as one who is functioning according to developmental norms with regard to gender expectations, who has established an age-appropriate sense of identity, and who has access to higher-level defenses normatively accepted for that age, especially as demonstrated by resourcefulness in the adaptive and flexible use of coping and defense mechanisms. Such a child can establish relationships with others, anticipate events, perform and complete academic and nonacademic tasks, and use humor and sublimation. The youngster's social relationships reflect a capacity for empathy and mutuality, a concern for others, and the ability to have true "buddies" and not mere casual friendships. The child can delay impulsive reactions and show the capacity for self-reflection and reality testing and a developed sense of reality. The child's identity includes sound super-ego functioning, reflected by a capacity to know rules, to learn from mistakes, to experience remorse, and to make reparations.

The components, described separately below, are best viewed as interacting contributors to a developing personality and to personality disorders.

TEMPERAMENT

Definition. The distinctions among temperament, emotions, and personality are not always clear. Some—and we include ourselves here—consider temperament to be a personality trait that appears very early in life (Hagekull 1994); others, when referring to traits such as timidity, assertiveness, and shyness, seem to use temperament and personality synonymously (see, for example, Plutchik 1993). Another example refers to the "core emotional organizations" in children (Magai and Hunziker 1993), which include such elements as "contentment" and "wary hostility," reminiscent of descriptions of such adult personality factors as "agreeableness" (Costa and McCrae 1994) and dimensions of temperament, such as "fear" (Rothbart et al. 1995). Temperament consensually refers to behaviors that appear early in life, usually during the first year—in other words, to behaviors likely to have biological and genetic origins, to have neurobiological correlates, and to be stable across situations and over time (Rutter 1987, Wachs 1994). Temperament contributes an emotional component to the formation and expression of personality. It is in the management of this emotionality over the course of development that temperament acts as a constant contributor to personality.

Measurement. The overlap in concepts and terms used to identify temperament, personality, and symptomatology in children occurs at least partly because they are all often measured in similar fashion. Typically, parents or teachers are given questionnaires and are asked to indicate the behaviors that characterize the child. The content of such questionnaires is dictated by the child's developmental level, which determines his behavioral capabilities. Changes in the content with age will reflect the greater impact of developing cognition and motivation and the more muted and less obvious impact of neurobiology. For example, by middle childhood, activity level (especially on teacher ratings) becomes a less obvious and less important personality characteristic (Eaton 1994).

Organization. Statistical approaches, such as factor analysis, are applied to questionnaire results to determine if there is a structure or organization that characterizes temperament. Several common factors have emerged from child temperament scales, including the seminal work of the New York Longitudinal Study (Thomas and Chess 1977). They are:

activity (e.g., speed and control of gross motor activity)

negative emotionality, including the intensity and frequency of negative reactions and their contributors (e.g., frustration, novelty, stress)

task persistence, which involves learning and attention and is more apparent in teacher ratings than in parent ratings

adaptability (i.e., to change), with the attendant self-management skills

inhibition, a robust scale that describes initial reactions to strangers and the tendency to seek or avoid novelty

biological rhythmicity and threshold, a factor more apparent in infants and preschoolers, which reflects the child's irritability in reaction to stimulation (Martin et al. 1994).

The five factors that emerged in the analysis of temperament inventories by A. Angleitner and F. Ostendorf (1994) were emotional stability, rhythmicity, activity and tempo, sociability, and impulse control.

Similar statistical approaches are used with personality scales, which also depend on a rater's response to lists of behaviors and qualities of personality. Children are rated by adult observers, whereas the results of adult personality scales are based on self-ratings. Analyses of adult personality questionnaires consistently identify five factors that characterize normal adult personality (Goldberg and Rosolack 1994). Paul Costa and Robert Mc-Crae (1998) have been instrumental in developing the Five-Factor Model (FFM), which may also be useful for understanding personality disorders (Costa and Widiger 1994). The five higher order or broad dimensions of the FFM, together with its associated facets or trait qualities, follow (Costa and McCrae 1994).

1. *Neuroticism* (N) refers to the individual's typical level of emotional adjustment. Individuals with high ratings on this dimension often experience psychological distress. Among its component facets are anxiety, angry hostility, depression, and vulnerability.
2. *Extraversion* (E) refers to the individual's need for stimulation, his preferred style of interpersonal interaction, and his experience of pleasure. High E individuals tend to be sociable, optimistic, and affectionate, whereas Low E individuals are more reserved, independent, and quiet but not necessarily unfriendly.
3. *Openness* (O) refers to an individual's curiosity and seeking of novelty. High O individuals are imaginative and may be unconventional, whereas Low E individuals are more conservative.
4. *Agreeableness* (A) refers to how individuals relate to others. High A individuals tend to be trusting, nurturant, and empathic, whereas Low A individuals (referred to as "antagonistic") tend to be cynical, suspicious, and irritable; they can be ruthless.
5. *Conscientiousness* (C) refers to an individual's organization and persistence when pursuing goals. High C individuals are organized, punctual, and persevering, whereas Low C individuals are more careless or lazy.

J. Digman (1994) has also reported that five factors can describe children's personality. Digman's factors are Extraversion, Friendliness, Conscientiousness, Neuroticism, and Intellect. They are remarkably similar to the FFM and suggest that there may be developmental continuity between the structure of personality in children and adults.

John and colleagues (1994) have also demonstrated that the FFM can be applied to adolescents, but they also note that there are important developmental differences. For example, they identified an "irritability" factor in the adolescents that is not seen as a separate entity in adults. They suggest that this finding may indicate that the factor of Neuroticism, of which irritability is a component, undergoes change with development, perhaps integrating components that were separate earlier in development.

When regarding the relationship between temperament and personality, it is worthy to note that when Digman (1994) removed those scale items that were related to Intellect, the resulting four factors were Sociability, Fear, Anger, and Impulsivity. These four factors are similar to the factors seen with child temperament scales. In effect, as the cognition that characterizes the developing child becomes more obvious to adults and is more easily measured on or reflected by questionnaires, the structure (or factors) of personality in children, adolescents, and adults appears to be more similar, and the distinction between temperament and personality becomes more apparent.

M. Rothbart and colleagues (1994, 1995) have offered a model of temperament that is useful in fostering integrative thinking about several of the components of personality. They define temperament as "constitutionally based individual differences in reactivity and self-regulation within the domains of emotionality, motor activity, and attention" (Rothbart et al. 1995, p. 315). They tried to identify psychological processes that underlie personality and, when possible, the neural systems that support these processes. This approach is distinguished from those like the Five-Factor Model, which statistically identifies dimensions of personality on the basis of behavioral similarities (Ahadi and Rothbart 1994). Derryberry and Rothbart (1997) recently presented an approach to viewing temperament as a possible precursor of personality by distinguishing between Motivational and Attentional Systems and their underlying neural substrates.

THE MOTIVATIONAL SYSTEM

According to D. Derryberry and M. Rothbart (1997), the Motivational System has evolved to serve positive approach, defensive, and nurturant needs and is controlled by the limbic system of the brain. It includes four types of behaviors: Approach, Fearful, Frustrative and Aggressive, and Affiliative and Nurturant.

1. *Approach behaviors* are those typically included under Extraversion. They involve sensitivity to rewards and active interaction with the environment, sociability in the attempt to obtain rewards from others, impulsivity in reacting to signals that rewards are possible, sensation seeking, and activity level. By six months of age, children are found to differ in smiling, laughing, and their latency to approach objects. Approach tendencies seen in infants are related to approach tendencies and impulsivity in 7-year-olds.

2. *Fearful behaviors* were referred to as anxiety systems in earlier versions of this model. They include expressions of fear, anger, and frustration; sadness; shyness; discomfort; and low ability to be soothed. These qualities, which can be seen by nine months of age, result in an inhibition of behavior, and they appear later in development than approach behaviors. Fearful inhibition is a stable characteristic, and significant correlations are found between infant fearfulness and toddler fearfulness and between early fearfulness and the kind that surfaces when the children are reevaluated at 7 years of age.

3. *Frustrative and Aggressive behaviors* have different correlates from fearful behaviors, so Derryberry and Rothbart (1997) argue that negative emotionality should be differentiated accordingly. Whereas fear in the very young is inversely related to positive emotionality at 6 to 7 years of age, frustration bears a direct relation to positive emotionality in that period. Also, infant fear predicts lower approach behavior, but infant anger or frustration predicts more approach behavior at 6 to 7 years of age. Frustration and anger may reflect approach behaviors that have failed because of delays or misunderstandings. Once the child is clearer in the expression of his needs, and if others are responsive, approach behaviors should emerge unhampered.

4. *Affiliative and Nurturant behaviors* encompass affectionate behaviors and may relate to the development of conscience, empathy, and altruism.

THE ATTENTIONAL SYSTEM

The Attentional System makes distinctions among different functions and associated cortical areas: a Vigilance System that maintains alertness and supports defensive behavior; a Posterior Attentional System that controls orienting functions and allows attention to disengage from one focus and reengage at another; and an Anterior (Cortical) System that includes executive functions that regulate the Posterior System, control attention to semantic information, and are basic to the effortful control afforded by such operations as planning and anticipation.

Derryberry and Rothbart (1997) have suggested many interesting implications of their model. For example, the child with strong approach tendencies will be exposed to a different world than that seen by the fearful, avoidant child: Specifically, the approach-oriented child will have exposure to more novel situations and moments and will experience positive affects during these experiences, whereas the fearful child will avoid novelty, seek familiarity, and experience negative affects in novel situations. Thus, their developing representations of themselves, others, and their world will be different. Some will be alert to danger, see danger where others see excitement, and see themselves as vulnerable rather than as competent and likable. (The absence of negative emotionality is not the ideal developmental goal, however, because negative emotionality is also related to the development of positive qualities, such as empathy and conscience. For some especially aggressive children, their minimal level of fear may leave them without a mechanism with which to modify their aggression.)

The model also has implications for treatment. Aside from the pharmacological implications of the cortical underpinnings of Approach and Anxiety Systems, Derryberry and Rothbart have suggested how children's attention may be shifted to help their adjustment. Avoidant children who rivet their attention on danger and escape may be helped to discover methods of coping and danger reduction by engagement rather than by flight; fearful children may be helped to direct their attention away from their bodily sensations.

Derryberry and Rothbart's work helps in conceptualizing the transition from temperament to personality and in thinking about clinical and practical applications. T. Wachs (1994) has emphasized the "fit" between the child's temperament and the environment. He has pointed out that a shy child can develop in the direction of either greater introversion and neuroticism or greater extroversion and stability, depending on the nature of the intervening environmental experiences. It is of interest and perhaps some irony that temperament models, which suggest such a strong genetic component, can provide one basis for conceptualizing interventions that modify the effect of temperamental extremes.

IDENTITY

Identity is not a simple, unitary concept. It has intrapsychic and interpersonal features (Akhtar and Samuel 1996) that were described in E. Erikson's seminal work (1959), which spoke of personal identity as an awareness by the individual of his "selfsameness and continuity in time" (p. 23) and also of others' recognition of this self-sameness and continuity in the individual.

Erikson said that identity consolidation was central to normal adolescent development, and considerable academic research that followed was devoted to theoretical elaboration (e.g., delineating stages and types of identity) and assessment of identity formation in adolescents and young adults (Blasi and Glodis 1995, Marcia 1966). The process of identity formation, according to Erikson, is one in which the adolescent synthesizes and sheds previous identifications and introjections so that an integrated personal identity results. The recognition and acceptance of that person by her community is an important part of the process. However, according to Erikson, acute identity confusion can result when an adolescent faces the "demand for his simultaneous commitment to physical intimacy, to decisive occupational choice, to energetic competition, and to psychosocial self-definition" (p. 166).

Identity, normal and pathological, is central to concepts of personality and personality disorder. S. Akhtar and S. Samuel (1996) have culled a number of components of identity from the literature that can prove useful for describing healthy identity and in guiding clinical interviewing and intervention. These components include realistic body image, subjective self-sameness, consistent attitudes and behaviors, temporal continuity of self-experience, genuineness and authenticity, gender clarity, internalized conscience, and ethnicity.

Object Relations theory describes an individual's internal, mental representation of self/other relationships. The individual's experience of her own identity is described in terms of her sense of separateness and individuation with regard to others. The integration of self- and other-representations undergoes a developmental process that is influenced by experiential and biological factors.

O. Kernberg (1976) has implicated identity diffusion as a core criterion of borderline personality organization. Identity diffusion refers to partial, rather than integrated, self- and other-representations that result from the use of defense mechanisms, such as splitting, that permit individuals to avoid awareness of the hated qualities in others whom they love and need. *DSM-IV* included identity disturbance ("markedly and persistently unstable self-image or sense of self," p. 654) as one of nine criteria for a borderline personality disorder (only five of which are needed for diagnosis). S. Hurt and colleagues (1992) have indicated that adult patients with a borderline personality disorder are a heterogeneous group; one subgroup, the Identity Cluster, is characterized by "chronic feelings of emptiness or boredom, identity disturbance, and intolerance of being alone" (pp. 201–202). Experiencing emptiness and difficulty being alone are also seen in preadolescent borderline children (Bleiberg 1994).

The preceding formulations emphasize a process of identity formation that accelerates during adolescence and reaches a resolution by young adulthood. It may be that identity—as defined by an ability to integrate some identifications and eliminate others and to employ an orientation to the future in order to conceptualize occupations and relationships—requires elements of the formal operational reasoning that emerges in adolescents (Inhelder and Piaget 1958).

Yet, although the concept of identity is clearly central to personality and its disorders, a formulation that restricts it to adolescent development limits its usefulness for those who work with preadolescents. The components described by Akhtar and Samuel (1996) and the features of the Identity Cluster identified by Hurt and colleagues (1992) can also be examined in children. Current research in developmental psychopathology rarely speaks of identity, but there is increasing emphasis on the child's development of the sense of self along with his developing awareness of the separate mental life of others. These increasingly sophisticated internal representations of self and other may be thought of as one way in which identity is manifested in younger children. Correspondingly, deviations in self- and other-representation can constitute the building blocks of personality disorders seen in adulthood.

By 18 months of age, normally developing children begin to demonstrate signs of recognition in front of a mirror (Lewis and Brooks-Gunn 1979), empathy toward others (and thereby distinguish between self and other [Hoffman 1977]), core gender identity (Stern 1985), and awareness of other's expectations or standards (Kagan 1991). The cognitive advances of middle childhood allow children to make comparisons between themselves and others by 6 to 7 years of age (Kagan 1991). Thus, the child's awareness and construction of the self and others appear early in development.

These mental structures are elaborated as the child grows, and they impact increasingly on her mental life and relationships with others. P. Fonagy and M. Target (1997) have described young children's competence to formulate and to act on their conception of others' beliefs, feelings, and plans, and they named this unconscious process "reflective function." Its development is related to the quality of the young child's interaction with his caregiver, especially the mother's mirroring or reflection of the child's state, which greatly influences the development of affect and its regulation. To illustrate, they described how mothers effectively soothe their 8-month-olds after an injection by rapidly mirroring the child's emotion but then mixing it with other affects, such as smiling and a mocking display. By providing an accurate but not overwhelming playback to the child, the mother may be serving as a model of adaptive emotional regulation while also helping to contain her baby's unpleasant affect state.

Fonagy and Target suggested that secure attachment results from successful containment by the mother, whereas insecure attachment is the result of the infant's identification with the mother's anxious, defensive behavior (p. 686). If these defenses are internalized, the child's own behaviors are not being clearly represented. The result can be a self that is constructed around a false internalization. Fonagy and Target have indicated that this may be a way to understand how a child with a PD comes to "feel a sense of alienation from their core self" (p. 696). In effect, a very young child can be seen to begin to develop features of the Identity Cluster characteristic of adults with severe borderline personality disorder.

Fonagy and Target also indicated possible relationships between attachment status, the child's sense of the other's mental life, and a sense of self. The secure infant can feel safe in making attributions about what thoughts account for his caregiver's behavior. The avoidant child, however, not only is behaviorally avoidant but also avoids the mental state of the other; the resistant child tends to focus only on his own state of distress. It is not hard to imagine children such as these going on to develop narcissistic or antisocial PDs characterized by a lack of empathy and an overfocusing on themselves. In addition, it is clear that secure attachment can foster cognitive development because the child has the luxury of being curious and of taking intellectual risks.

Children with disorganized attachment may have to be overly aware of the mother's behavior and intentional states: they cannot afford errors in predicting caregiver behavior. Because they must expend so much of their energy and thought on understanding their parents rather than on reflecting freely on their own self-states (Fonagy and Target 1997), the complexity and organization of their own selves may suffer.

Thus, children who have been traumatized are less likely to develop a style that allows them to think clearly about their mental state, especially during stressful interactions, because they are so vigilant about the other. Because this style dominates more of traumatized children's relationships, Fonagy and Target have suggested that an adult PD can ensue. Consistent with their suggestion is the finding by M. Patrick and colleagues (1994), who used the AAI with borderline adults (as contrasted with dysthymic controls) and found that the borderline patients were confused and did not have an integrated mental framework for containing and thinking about their early experiences.

R. S. Wallerstein (1998) has pointed out that in current psychoanalytic thinking, identity maintains a position of importance, but it is expressed in terms of the self. This perspective is useful for several reasons. Traditionally, identity is so firmly linked to adolescence that thinking about it in the context of younger children is constrained. Conceptualizations of the self, on the other hand, foster elaborations about self/other representations, the development of affect, and the contribution of attachment relationships, all of which can potentially be assessed as the child develops. These elements are found to relate, in turn, to the child's social behavior, self-esteem, sense of efficacy in his world, and other features that are relevant for diagnosing PDs because self-representations can constitute the more enduring features of the child's mental life.

GENDER

Gender is a fundamental dimension around which children identify themselves. It influences how others react toward them, and it needs to be thought about in the evaluation of each child. Gender identity is established by 2 years of age as a self-construct around which children consistently organize themselves and their activities. Gender identity disorders can be observed in children, manifested in different, characteristic ways in boys and girls (*DSM-IV*).

Longitudinal research has demonstrated that gender is an important individual difference variable. J. Block (1993) indicated that gender is related to children's adaptations before and after divorce and that it modifies the relationship between childhood qualities and later behaviors, such as drug use and the exhibition of depressive tendencies. Block (1993) reported that the relationship between ego-resiliency and ego-control over time is different for boys and girls. Namely, adaptation to the changes of adolescence, as reflected by the construct of ego-resiliency, may require more restructuring for girls than for boys. For girls to abandon the previous, more restrictive modes of adaptation of childhood requires resiliency and a movement away from overcontrol.

NEUROPSYCHOLOGICAL DEVELOPMENTAL DISORDERS

Two neuropsychological patterns illustrate how cognitive features need to be considered when evaluating children. (They should also be considered when evaluating adults; they reflect one way in which child evaluations and psychopathology can inform work with adults.) These features also contribute to integrative thinking about temperament, identity, and personality development.

The first of these neuropsychological patterns is the executive function deficit found in children with Attention Deficit Hyperactivity Disorder (ADHD) (Pennington and Ozonoff 1996). Executive functions include the abilities to plan, to inhibit, to self-monitor, and to deploy effectively working memory. In effect, executive functions influence how a child plans to carry out a particular action, to hold in mind certain plans or actions until the right time to carry them out in the behavioral or problem-solving sequence, to inhibit irrelevant actions, and to self-monitor his work as he moves along. R. Barkley (1997) has argued that ADHD is, furthermore, associated with executive function impairments in working memory, behavioral inhibition, regulation of motivation, and motor control. Executive function deficits are also seen in children with learning disabilities in reading and mathematics.

Derryberry and Rothbart's (1997) model of temperament includes an Attentional System that controls other systems and that relies on the successful deployment of executive functions. Temperamental difficulties, therefore, may also bring with them hard-wired executive dysfunction. It also seems likely that the child who is temperamentally difficult, who cannot inhibit behaviors, who cannot reflect on what he has done or cannot anticipate consequences for his actions, is impacting parental input and thus contributing to potentially insecure attachments, which in turn can affect the development of executive functions. It is not surprising that secure attachment is a good predictor of metacognitive ability in memory, comprehension, and communication (Moss et al. 1995).

The behavioral tendencies that reflect the contribution of a difficult temperament, derived from frontal lobe dysfunction, may also affect the development of a sense of self by constraining parental reactions and by influencing the child's capacity to attend to and to integrate parental behaviors and affects. Interventions that employ cognitive behavioral strategies in the older child therefore may not only teach him new scripts that allow for more differentiated self/other representations but may also help foster verbal control of behavior, self-reflection, and planning—the very steps that are deficient in PDs characterized by impulse control deficits.

It is not surprising, then, that some adults with a borderline personality disorder have shown evidence of organicity, such as hyperactivity and minimal brain dysfunction, earlier terms for ADHD (Andrulonis et al. 1980).

The second neuropsychological pattern is the nonverbal learning disability syndrome, as described by B. Rourke (1989). People with this problem produce much higher verbal IQ scores than performance IQ scores. They exhibit good word decoding but poor reading comprehension, difficulty with mathematics, and a concreteness or literalness that would not be expected on the basis of their verbal intellectual ability.

In terms of personality, they are characterized by deficits in reading social cues, perspective-taking, social judgment, and social interaction skills. The children seen with this pattern, in line with Rourke's description, are described as shy and withdrawn from peers. They face their greatest problems in group situations where the demands for rapid information processing and give-and-take are greatest; they do much better with one other person.

Thus, these children present a syndrome that is consistent with an avoidant PD—but this syndrome may represent a continuum because adults who demonstrate a schizoid PD also display this psychometric pattern. (For example, a 33-year-old male with the cognitive and learning features just described, who had not been able to complete college, said that he could not understand why his roommates were angry with him for eating and not replacing all the food they put in the refrigerator.) Children and adults with these PDs and this learning syndrome require cognitive as well as psychotherapeutic intervention, which may involve social skills training and training in metacognitive skills.

The foregoing neuropsychological patterns, which might be termed frontal and right hemisphere patterns, indicate the central role that organic deficits can play in the development of some PDs. They also demonstrate that a careful cognitive evaluation of children and adults can contribute important information to the evaluation of, and treatment planning for, PDs.

DEFENSE MECHANISMS

Freud (1936) suggested that a person selects from among the variety of available defense mechanisms, which then become an intrinsic aspect of his character. They are reevoked in situations that resemble the original one, and the person may actually seek or induce situations that could justify their use. For example, a child who has been physically abused and becomes identified with the aggressor repeats actively the abuse he experienced passively, paving the way for the development of a sadistic trait.

R. S. Wallerstein (1983) has distinguished between defense mechanisms and defensive behaviors. Defense mechanisms, which are theoretical explanatory constructs, are functions of the mind that are used in combination to explain observable defensive behaviors, affects, and ideas. Following Vaillant (1977) and C. Perry and colleagues (1993), among others, P. F. Kernberg (1994) has proposed a list of defense mechanisms that include:

the normal defenses that characterize normal personality (e.g., humor, suppression, sublimation);

the neurotic defenses that correlate with the neurotic personality organization (e.g., repression, undoing, projection, isolation, turning against the self, intellectualization, rationalization);

the borderline defenses that correlate with borderline personality organization, that is, histrionic, borderline, narcissistic, and antisocial personality disorders (e.g., splitting, denial, idealization, devaluation, projective identification, acting out); and

the psychotic defense mechanisms that correlate with the psychotic personality organization, that is, schizotypal, hypomanic, and paranoid personality disorders (e.g., de-animation, hypochondriasis, constriction, fusion, autistic encapsulation).

M. J. Horowitz and colleagues (1990) have given a cognitive definition to defense mechanisms by relating them to cognitive operations outside of the awareness of the person. These cognitive controls organize thoughts and feelings. Another type of control or defense determines the sequence of feelings and ideas typical for each individual's personality style, be it normal or pathological.

The understanding of defensive behaviors as clusters of defense mechanisms fosters the development of psychotherapeutic approaches. Personality consists of behaviors that have become automatic and are structured in the personality so that their rate of change is slow because they have now become traits and are no longer transitory states. Psychoanalytic psychotherapies, by making the person aware of the maladaptive impact of his defenses on his functioning, permit the resolution of these clusters of defense mechanisms, one by one, so as to render them obsolete. Indeed, the patient can resolve severe pathology by replacing primitive defenses with more mature ones. Vaillant (1977) has been most persuasive in pointing to the correlation of level of defenses with social and professional adaptation, academic and professional success, marital and parenting capacities, and physical morbidity and mortality.

AFFECTS

According to Vaillant (1977), the affective component in a person's expression reflects the efficiency of his mechanisms of defense. Indeed, the capacities to express and to verbalize a full range of affects toward others and to move smoothly from one affect to another may correspond to the use of more mature defense mechanisms, as seen in people with normal or neurotic personality organization. In contrast, people with severe PD or borderline personality organization are characterized by a restricted spectrum of affects that are more in the dysphoric range, that show limited modulation within the same affect, and that move abruptly from one affect to another. Primitive, borderline defenses based on splitting mechanisms are in operation here. When affects are inappropriate to content, a psychotic personality organization is present, along with its corresponding psychotic defense mechanisms (schizotypal, hypomanic, paranoid).

Those with borderline personality organization illustrate how affect also plays a role in forming the link between mental representations of self and other. For example, a 33-year-old woman constantly spoke in her therapy sessions about her anger at her father. When asked what would happen if she stopped being angry at him, she said, "He would die." Her father had been dead for many years, but retaining her anger allowed her to keep his representation alive.

CONCLUSION

Each personality disorder represents the end point of a complicated biopsychosocial process. "Real life" is even more complicated because so many children and adults who have a PD also have co-occurring PDs. The clinician evaluating and planning treatment for a child or an adolescent is well advised to examine each of the personality components previously described, and to especially consider the interactions and interweaving of these variables. By so doing, the clinician can consider the child simultaneously as the object and as the agent of formative input.

PART II
ASSESSMENT OF PERSONALITY DISORDERS IN CHILDREN AND ADOLESCENTS

II.1

Assessment of Personality Disorders in Children and Adolescents

This chapter presents a two-pronged clinical approach to the evaluation of PDs in children and adolescents as evidenced by both *behavioral patterns* descriptive of specific PDs and *structural characteristics* underlying basic personality organizations. A reliance on descriptive characteristics alone can be misleading: The behaviors associated with hysterical PD (neurotic personality organization), for example, are similar to those associated with histrionic PD (borderline personality organization); avoidant PD (neurotic organization) superficially resembles schizoid PD (borderline organization). Likewise, differentiation may be made among obsessive PD patients functioning with neurotic, borderline, and psychotic organizations. Indeed, the very concept of personality organization permits an integrated view of the different components of personality—in other words, not as isolated behaviors but as elements rooted in a matrix greater than the sum of its individual traits.

The chart below (Figure IIa) outlines the general diagnostic criteria for a personality disorder as identified by *DSM-IV*. The criteria can be applied to the assessment of PDs in children, with the one modification that onset must be traced at least to the early school years, in keeping with the basic definition of PDs as enduring maladaptive patterns of thinking, feeling, and behavior that are relatively stable over time.

For the age ranges addressed in this book, it is important to distinguish persistent maladaptive patterns from those that are limited to a particular development stage; 2-year-olds, for example, are expected to be oppositionally defiant. Other than that alertness to age-specific behavior as *DSM-IV* states, there is no clear distinction between childhood and adult disorders (p. 37), and diagnostic categories are applicable to any individual—child or adult—who meets the criteria (p. 633).

Although this chapter underlines the categorical approach to the assessment of personality, it also makes reference to dimensional perspectives that yield other descriptors about an individual. Those dimensional perspectives encompass traits characteristic of everyone to varying degrees (e.g., extroversion/introversion, optimism/pessimism, assertiveness/shyness, impulsivity/control); temperamental traits are included as well. Variations in and among traits as dimensions of personality become more relevant in the normal personality or the neurotic organization. Severity is measured by the intensity and number of criteria involved. The coloring of a particular personality disorder derives from the braiding of dimensional criteria with the group of traits clustered categorically: Cluster A, odd-eccentric; Cluster B, dramatic-emotional; and Cluster C, anxious-fearful.

The assessment of an Axis II disorder is best made if the Axis I disorder is in remission (Brent et al. 1990). In other words, a narcissistic PD may surface only after a school phobia has been treated; an antisocial PD may emerge after an obsessive-compulsive disorder has been treated. Axis II shows high comorbidity with both affective disorder and with other Axis II disorders (6 to 15 percent). The recognition of an Axis II PD allows the clinician to formulate a more comprehensive treatment plan and to better evaluate responses to psychopharmacological agents because the presence of a PD worsens the overall prognosis and complicates the response to drugs. One 11-year-old boy treated for an obsessive-compulsive disorder with a combination of drug therapy, high doses of Prozac, and cognitive therapy met all criteria for an antisocial PD once his obsessive constriction improved. Ultimately, full discovery and acknowledgment of a patient's entire personality will improve his alliance and compliance with treatment.

Three forms of assessment will be described and illustrated in the pages that follow. Although each may produce both descriptive and structural information, we introduce them in the context of their primary targets: History-taking via questionnaires completed by family and others close to the patient yield descriptions of behavior patterns; interviewing the patient

FIGURE IIa   Diagnostic Criteria for a Personality Disorder

A.   An enduring pattern of inner experience and behavior that deviates markedly from the expectations of the individual's culture. This pattern is manifested in two (or more) of the following areas:

    (1)   cognition (i.e., ways of perceiving and interpreting self, other people, and events)
    (2)   affectivity (i.e., the range, sensitivity, lability, and appropriateness of emotional response)
    (3)   interpersonal functioning
    (4)   impulse control

B.   The enduring pattern is inflexible and pervasive across a broad range of personal and social situations.
C.   The enduring pattern leads to clinically significant distress or impairment in social, occupational, or other important areas of functioning.
D.   The pattern is stable and of long duration and its onset can be traced back at least to adolescence or early adulthood.
E.   The enduring pattern is not better accounted for as a manifestation or consequence of another mental disorder.
F.   The enduring pattern is not due to the direct physiological effects of a substance (e.g., a drug of abuse, a medication) or a general medical condition (e.g., head trauma)

Reproduced with permission DSM-IV.

(or observing his play) and psychological testing are the forums for structural insights.

ASSESSING DESCRIPTIVE CHARACTERISTICS: DEVELOPMENTAL HISTORY

In the patient's history, we look for indicators of high risk for the development of PDs—for example, such traumatic events as abuse, not only sexual and physical but also verbal abuse, which is known to be significantly more intense in the case of borderline PDs. The incidence of neglect, along with inconsistent parenting, seems to be more characteristic of antisocial PDs. Disturbed peer relationships evidencing possessiveness and omnipotent control are early characteristics of borderline personality organization; exploitativeness signals the antisocial personality. Hypersensitivity to interpersonal stresses, boredom, and devaluation distinguish narcissistic PDs. Histrionic personalities will have a history of dramatic affective expression and constant demands for attention through seductiveness. Problems of shyness and severe difficulties in making friends are common to avoidant personalities. Patients with obsessive-compulsive PDs manifest significant constriction during leisure activities; perfectionism, rigidity, and stubbornness are all present. Dependent PDs must be assessed against the developmentally appropriate dependent needs of children. Patterns of explosive temper, poor academic functioning, shifting levels of ego functioning, and impulsiveness are all clues to the clinician to undertake a personality assessment; without it, there will be no way to detect the beginning of a PD in childhood.

Many practitioners think it important when assessing PDs to obtain information from sources other than the patient (Tyrer 1991). The assessment of children typically requires contact with the adults around the child. Well-researched questionnaires have been designed to gather information from parents and teachers. For example, T. M. Achenbach's Child Behavior Checklist (CBCL) (1991) has been used in a range of studies and has provided valuable epidemiological information as well as data about specific disorders, such as Attention Deficit Disorder and anxiety disorders (Biederman 1992). While the syndromes and problem behavior areas identified presumably relate to Axis I mental disorders, many items in the questionnaires correspond to personality trait characteristics and can therefore apply to Axis II diagnoses. Categorical diagnosis as outlined in the *DSM-IV* system accounts for 49 percent of the variance of people with maladaptive traits (Loranger et al. 1994); the rest of that population may have up to 10 trait disorders that may not meet criteria for a categorical type but have enough intensity to produce impairments. Because children are in the process of development, we assume that not meeting full criteria but having several maladaptive traits is more likely to be the case among them. This area requires further research. Indeed, 57 percent of the questions on the Achenbach CBCL relate to personality traits considered by *DSM-IV* as criteria for some of the categorical PDs when construed as enduring and inflexible patterns.

The theoretical framework influences the manner in which behaviors are viewed and the conclusions that are drawn about PDs. The Achenbach CBCL offers a statistical perspective on individual behaviors that, by factor analysis, are grouped into two broad-band dimensions: Internalizing Disorders and Externalizing Disorders. The two higher-order factors subsume eight subfactors, among which are Withdrawn, Anxious/Depressed, and Social Problems (all Internalizing), and Attention Problems, Delinquent Behavior, and Aggressive Behavior (all Externalizing). These CBCL items reflect particular PDs as they are described in the literature and are presented in *DSM-IV*.

Others reveal enduring qualities characteristic of PDs in general. These same components can be independently assessed in psychological testing.

What follows is a regrouping of Achenbach's behavior checklist in terms of PD criteria. The numbers between parentheses refer to the numbered items in the Achenbach's behavior checklist.

BORDERLINE PERSONALITY DISORDER

Argues a lot (3)

Complains of loneliness (12)

Cruelty, bullying, or meanness to others (16)

Deliberately harms self or attempts suicide (18)

Destroys his or her own things (20)

Feels or complains that no one loves him or her (33)

Impulsive or acts without thinking (41)

Physically attacks other people (57)

Screams a lot (68)

Sudden changes in mood or feelings (87)

Talks about killing self (91)

Temper tantrums or hot temper (95)

NARCISSISTIC PERSONALITY DISORDER

Bragging and boasting (7)

Disobedient at home (22)

Disobedient at school (23)

Feels he or she has to be perfect (32)

Showing off or clowning (74)

ANTISOCIAL PERSONALITY DISORDER

Cruel to animals (15)

Cruelty, bullying, or meanness to others (16)

Destroys things belonging to his or her family or others (21)

Doesn't seem to feel guilty after misbehaving (26)

Gets in many fights (37)

Impulsive or acts without thinking (41)

Lying or cheating (43)

Runs away from home (67)

Sets fires (72)

Steals at home (81)

Steals outside the home (82)

Threatens people (97)

Truancy, skips school (101)

Vandalism (106)

HISTRIONIC PERSONALITY DISORDER

Demands a lot of attention (19)

Interaction with others is often characterized by inappropriate sexually seductive or provocative behavior (73)

PARANOID PERSONALITY DISORDER

Easily jealous (27)

Feels others are out to get him or her (34)

Secretive, keeps things to himself or herself (69)

Suspicious (89)

SCHIZOID PERSONALITY DISORDER

Would rather be alone than with others (22)

Doesn't get along with other kids (25)

Strange behaviors (84)

Withdrawn, doesn't get involved with others (111)

Strange ideas (85)

AVOIDANT PERSONALITY DISORDER

Fears he or she might think or do something bad (31)

Self-conscious or easily embarrassed (71)

Shy or timid (75)

DEPENDENT PERSONALITY DISORDER

Acts too young for his or her age (1)   Whining (109)

Clings to adults or is too dependent (11)

Stores up things that he or she does not need (83)

Stubborn, sullen, or irritable (86)

Too concerned with meekness or cleanliness (99)

GENERAL PERSONALITY DISORDER TRAITS

Feels worthless or inferior (35)

Gets hurt a lot, accident prone (36)

Gets teased a lot (38)

Hangs around with others who get in trouble (39)

Nervous, high strung, or tense (45)

Not liked by other kids (48)

Too fearful or anxious (50)

Poorly coordinated or clumsy (62)

Prefers being with older kids (63)

Prefers being with younger kids (64)

Sulks a lot (88)

Talks too much (93)

Teases a lot (94)

Thinks about sex too much (96)

Worries (112)

ASSESSING STRUCTURAL CHARACTERISTICS: THE INTERVIEW

Identity

Identity is one of the central concepts in the area of personality and personality disorders. As defined by E. Erikson (1959), it refers to the sense of continuity within oneself and in terms of one's interactions with others. Identity reflects the awareness of one's individuality and one's allegiance to the ideology and culture of his group (Erikson 1959). It implies a sense of purpose, intentionality, and mastery.

Components of Identity

Akhtar and Samuel (1996), in a review of the concept of identity, concluded that identity originates in the earliest exchanges between the infant and her mother and develops throughout the life cycle. Although in adolescence there is a remodeling of the components of identity, further development does continue during young adulthood, mid-life, and later years.

Descriptively, identity relates to the following features, according to Akhtar and Samuel:

- A realistic body image. The person is anchored in her own body, recognizes herself in a mirror, is capable of making reasonable estimates of her weight, appearance, and body size, and displays resilience even in the face of physical changes, such as pregnancy or alterations resulting from an accident.

- Subjective self-sameness. The person experiences himself to be the same across situations. He can adapt to different circumstances or different age groups with flexibility and without losing internal constancy (self-constancy).
- Consistent attitudes and behaviors. The person has the capacity for a stable investment in values and ideologies. Behavior is congruent with what she is and how she behaves. Even among different forms of expression in the repertoire of the integrated identity, there is flexibility for smooth transitions between the various self-representations emerging under diverse social circumstances.
- Temporal continuity. There is a sense of personal continuity across time. The person has the capacity to recognize himself as the same person from childhood to adolescence and to project himself into the future.
- Authenticity. The person has a true capacity to recognize the positive and negative traits that make her genuinely herself. In contrast with the concept of pseudo-self that has been described as a premature closure and a primitive identification with others, authenticity refers to selective identifications with important figures in one's life. It means being fully genuine, sincere, and trustworthy.
- Gender. Gender identity consists of the awareness of being male or female (core gender identity), the awareness of one's femininity or masculinity (gender role), and one's sexual orientation (heterosexual or homosexual). Thus a cohesive gender identity betokens harmony between core gender identity, gender role, and sexual orientation. In children, the distinction between the sexes and the awareness of irreversibility of core gender are achievements of the third and fourth year of life. Play characteristics, fantasies, dress patterns, and friendship patterns are revealing, as in the assumption of feminine roles by boys with gender identity disorder, or in their preference for girls as friends with whom to identify.
- Ethnicity. Ethnicity relates to the values, child-rearing practices, culture, language and nonverbal modes of expression, and patterns of interpersonal behavior with which the child grows up. Ethnic identity is formed through language, through traditions, and through the feeling of belonging to the historical community and national community.
- Superego or conscience. The person has the capacity to respond to rewards and punishments; to experience remorse, guilt, and shame; to wish to atone for damage done; and to work for ideals. Concern for

others and generosity are personality traits reflecting an integrated conscience.

Akhtar and Samuel summarized the postadolescent identity as incorporating a realistic body image, sustained self-sameness, a certain consistency of attitudes and behavior, temporal continuity in the self-experience, genuineness and authenticity, clarity regarding one's gender, an inner solidarity with an ethnic group's ideals, and internalized conscience.

In our opinion, school-aged children and adolescents can also meet these criteria. The child with an integrated identity conveys a sense of "meness"—that is, a sense of a cohesive self in its positive and negative aspects, of boundaries and autonomy, of continuity across time and situations. He expresses his sense of belonging to a family and an ethnic or religious group. He displays moral and ethical values and an ego ideal that reveals an internalized conscience—a mature superego that monitors his thoughts and actions and rewards or punishes with guilt feelings. Thus, the child can compare himself with an ideal that by and large is within his reach.

Identity Crisis and Identity Diffusion

Identity crisis relates to the discrepancy between rapidly shifting physical and psychological selves, complete with sexual impulses; a widening gap occurs between self-perception and the experiences of others' perceptions (O. Kernberg 1978). In contrast, identity diffusion refers to the lack of integration of the concept of self and significant others whereby the clinician cannot form a picture of the patient's vision of himself or other important people in his life. There is a lack of resolution of the stage of separation/individuation in the sense that object constancy and self-constancy are not achieved. The pathology, relatively less evident at school age, tends to break through in adolescence with the loosening of external social structures. Identity diffusion appears as chaotic self-description; descriptions of others are full of contradictory statements and rigid clichés. The person looks indecisive and undefined or relatively affectless or pseudo-submissive, as in the quiet borderline PD (Sherwood 1994, P. Kernberg and Koenigsberg 1999).

The superego in identity diffusion does not become integrated into a conscience but remains fixed in its precursors—that is, in persecutory superego imagoes that leave the child's mind with terrifying anxieties of engulfing destruction and invasiveness. Group activities are undertaken under the shadow of charismatic leaders from whom the individual derives a borrowed identity in place of an autonomous one. Much group gang psychology can be explained along these lines. Lying and deceitfulness in children must be explored in terms of identity diffusion as well as in terms of superego functioning. Tactfully confronting lies will reveal no remorse or guilt; indeed, the child's incapacity to empathize with the ethical values of the culture or with the interviewer supports the likelihood of a diagnosis of narcissistic or antisocial personality disorder.

Assessing Identity

In the clinical interview, identity can be either described by the adolescent or child or demonstrated in the actual behaviors, verbal and nonverbal, in the interaction with the examiner. The adolescent can be asked such questions as, Can you tell me about yourself? your religion? your ethnic background? how you see yourself physically? What are you like? How do you see yourself in the mirror? How would you deal with changing circumstances? with different people? Can you predict your attitudes and behaviors? How do you feel about the changes within yourself?

Friendships enhance one's identity, including gender identity, and the description of friendships can be significant (P. Kernberg, A. Clarkin, et al. 1992). There is a difference between a normal 9-year-old who describes his friend as someone nice to be with ("She can be stubborn and we fight, but we always make up") and a child with antisocial PD who cannot describe his friend except by saying that "He has a lot of Ninja Turtles and computer games and a water mattress." If an older child or adolescent can describe not only himself in his complexity (positive and negative qualities) but also his family and friends, if he is able to relate to others as independent individuals and not as possessions or extensions of himself, he is likely to have a more integrated identity.

Self- and Other-Representations

In a structural sense, identity, the subjective component of personality, is the product of the integration of self-representation and object- (i.e., other-) representations connected by affective links and language.

How the person describes and reflects upon himself, how he interacts and empathizes with the interviewer, how he expresses himself verbally, and how he expresses his affects will tell us what he is like—that is, will articulate the identity and personality organization that will be evoked and observed. Cognitive and affective styles (self- and object-representations, observing ego, and self-reflective empathy with the interviewer's intentions and purposes) are basic components of personality and will emerge during clinical interviews.

THE PERSONALITY ASSESSMENT INTERVIEW

Components of personality can be assessed by means of different interviewing techniques. The Personality Assessment Interview (PAI), developed by M. Selzer, Paulina Kernberg, and colleagues (1987), demonstrates personality function in a focused way in terms of these variables: self- and object-representations, cognition, affects, reflective capacity or observing ego, and empathy with the interviewer. The 45-minute PAI was derived from the structural interview developed by O. Kernberg (1988), whose underlying hypothesis is that the patient's experience of the interview taps into his fantasies and influences his style of interaction with the examiner. The interview is conceived to elicit the basic components of the personality and its governing principles of organization and coping.

The PAI technique consists of systematically asking questions that involve self-representation, object-representation, ego observation, and empathy, observing affect and cognitions as the patient talks. At 5- to 10-minute intervals, the interviewer asks:

[First loop] *What have you been told about this interview with me?*

[Second loop] *Now that we have been together, how does what happened compare with your initial impressions?*

[Third loop] *Now that we have spent x minutes together, what do you expect the rest of the meeting to be like?*

[Fourth loop] *What have you learned about the interview, about yourself, and about me, and what do you imagine I have understood so far?*

[Fifth loop] *What do you expect the end of the meeting to be?*

Meanwhile, the interviewer is probing, Who are you? what are you like? who are they? what are they like? who am I? what am I like? what are you doing? and, what am I doing? She creates repeated opportunities to observe self-representations, object-representations, affects, cognition, ego observations, and empathy and will be equipped to acquire a good impression of each variable.

The PAI seems particularly well suited for adolescents, who are generally reluctant to talk to adults about their personal history. This interview does not inquire about their private lives. One patient commented, "I think you have been interested not only in the answers to your questions, but in me." Assessment of adolescents' experience of the interview has found that the subjects do not find the interviewer intrusive; moreover, they welcome intensity of the interaction and feel that the interviewer is listening to them attentively.

The PAI helps to assess the capacity of the adolescent for psychotherapy because it taps such functions crucial to the success of the process as attention, memory, capacity for reflection, and capacity for a therapeutic alliance. The patient's capacity to observe himself in the interaction and to observe the process of the interview can yield a persuasive measure of the patient's reality testing. One adolescent said, "We are going around and around in this and wasting our time. This is only a conversation about a conversation."

It is interesting to see how adolescents who look objectively similar can appear quite different under the prism of this interview. This distinction was true of two inpatients who were very close friends. One was the president of the patient group and the other her secretary; both were thought to be nearly ready to end their treatment in the unit. The first patient performed at the highest levels of our scales on the six dimensions, but the second clearly showed confusion and a lack of differentiation in her sense of self and her perceptions of others. The staff was shocked to see such a difference in these two girls; the second resembled an "as-if" personality, taking on the colors of her friend and appearing healthier than she was.

What follows are excerpts from a PAI with a 17-year-old youth (white, Protestant) who had a history of poor conduct, including cutting classes, running away from home, fighting with his father, and engaging in multiple substance abuse (marijuana and cocaine, in addition to alcohol). At one point he had stolen his mother's jewels to pay his drug debts and had allowed the family maid to be blamed for the theft. He reported periods of social withdrawal, inactivity, sleep disturbance, and decreased energy level with intermittent emotional lability, suggesting depression. His father, an active businessman, was described as rigid, undemonstrative, and distant. His mother was seductive and infantalizing toward him; she herself suffered from periods of depression. A younger sibling suffered from various somatic complaints.

Psychological testing indicated a borderline personality organization with unmodulated affect, impulsivity, primitive defenses, fleeting constriction, and avoidance. Also evident were antisocial traits, such as rebelliousness against authority, proneness to self-serving acts with lack of empathy, and use of a false façade to manipulate others' impressions. In addition, there were deficits in his thought organization, with poor abstraction and difficulties in word finding. From the beginning of the interview, it was difficult for him to be specific and to respond to questions referring to himself.

THERAPIST: We will be talking about how you and I are relating to each other today, and maybe you can tell me a little about your expectations of meeting me today. What did you anticipate on your way?

PATIENT: Well, this is my tenth month here in the hospital; and a good portion of these ten months is I mean it's been a long time for me to really recognize my problems and really see what I have to work on. Now I'm really hoping that through this interview really you might help my doctor in ways of treating me, 'cause I really want work with my problems it's just very difficult, because I have a lot of things against me. And, that's really all and I really don't want to get left

[Notice the tendency to generalize, to be evasive.]

THERAPIST: So you have two kinds of problems: the ones that you came with, and then you are telling me that the staff who is working with you—they have problems in helping you.

PATIENT: Yeah. I think they do.

THERAPIST: Can you give me some examples of your own problems and the problems that you see with staff in helping you?

PATIENT: Well, I have difficulties in feeling . . . in dealing with sadness and anger. These emotions–I–as I try, I really never express them and I just kind of was a recluse in a way. Never really expressed them that much. And over the years I never really expressed them and it just mounted up until now, and I started acting on them impulsively and I am here to control that impulsivity and to work and deal with my feelings and it's really difficult. And what's really preventing me from really dealing with all these emotions are these deviancies that have built up over the years.

THERAPIST: These deviancies?

PATIENT: Yeah.

THERAPIST: What is that?

PATIENT: Er . . . psychological blocks that protect these feelings. Most of the time when I talk to people, I quickly edit what I say to them. I'm very careful what I say to people.

THERAPIST: Are you being careful right now, for example?

PATIENT: Er . . . I probably am. But not so much. I . . . I don't feel really strong at all. I feel very weak. I have . . . I've been experiencing a lot of these emotions lately and I feel scared—you know and it's really frustrating. I know it's a long road, you know, but it is something you gotta deal with.

THERAPIST: In the way that you are telling this to me, do you think that I have some . . . er . . . I am getting an idea of what you are going through with what you are telling me?

PATIENT: I think so. It's really difficult for me to show people what I'm feeling, 'cause if I did, I'd be a wreck.

THERAPIST: Well, today you came in and you told me that you were anxious about coming but you recognized that because your body tensed up. So you see you could tell me what you are feeling.

[At this point, the therapist reminds him of his capacity to observe himself, at least in terms of body feelings. At another point, he shows his splitting in his sense of self.]

THERAPIST: So you think that you are trying to appear a strong person.

PATIENT: Well—an all together person, you know. I have a lot of things going for me.

THERAPIST: But this is something that you will try to be or try to project . . .

PATIENT: Yeah, try to project to people.

THERAPIST: You mentioned just a couple of minutes ago that you feel rather weak. Can you tell me, then, in what ways you feel weak and in what ways you feel you have to appear strong?

PATIENT: Well.

THERAPIST: With relation to me right now, for example, you could tell me how you are handling the two feelings that you have . . . that you want to appear strong and then you want to appear weak.

[When confronted the patient is unable to respond and talks about his parents instead. Eventually he talks about his meekness, his fear, and his feelings.]

PATIENT: My parents are far away right now and I'm very close to my mother and close to my dad but it doesn't really show. I love my mom to the world . . . I'd do anything for her, and she's really . . . she is a strong support in me—you know, while I'm in here and having her 3,500 miles away makes me feel very nervous. I feel all alone, and she can't bail me out in these circumstances or do anything for me and I feel very much left alone and scary and it has caused me to feel a little sadness and anger recently and that's why I feel meek . . . I mean really meek, you know. It's just really difficult for me to cope with things these days.

THERAPIST: Only these days?

PATIENT: Basically these days. 'Cause these emotions are coming up in me all the time now, and it's hell to just really sit down and function and go to school and everything at the same time.

THERAPIST: You know, I asked you the question as to whether here with me you were feeling weak and you . . .

PATIENT: Yeah, I do.

THERAPIST: And you answered this about your mother. What do you think of that?

PATIENT: Well, I think it could be I didn't really want to answer your question so I gave you a different answer.

PATIENT: (when confronted, the patient shows his insight but only in a fleeting way). I kind of side-tracked . . . where there is a connection with my mother into that question. It's really difficult, you know, when someone asks me a question and I sidetrack, it's really difficult for me to, you know, look back and say, you know . . . well, what happened just there? So so I really can't say.

THERAPIST: And what did you consider your major flaws that you still have to work on?

PATIENT: I feel that I had begun to work on expressing my feelings. It's just that there is a lot more to—that I have to work on . . . on it a lot more and its going to be very painful. And it's extremely difficult because at the same time I feel that I'm manipulating my own defenses that are trying to protect these feelings.

[Therapist asserts that she is still unclear about what his specific problems are.]

PATIENT: Yeah, that's very true. It's funny you would say that. Recently in therapy there are times when I would really confuse my therapist about what I'm trying to say to him. And he's told me recently that there are times when he's not really sure if I am telling the truth or not and . . .

THERAPIST: What is it that you are doing that you communicated that to me so fast, you think?

PATIENT: Well, it's really—it's hard for me to talk to someone about my problems when I'm not really sure I'm telling the truth or not. I have a lot of ambivalence in me and I think that really affects how pure what I say is, true or not. Only it's rather difficult for me to talk to people because my problems are so complex and so interwebbed with other things. It's really hard to really know what's right and what's wrong. And what I say to people all the time is as clear as I understand about what my problems are at the time or my opinion or my thoughts about them, but my life changes . . .

THERAPIST: You know, I think when I told you that you were kind of trying to see whether you could get away with what you are talking—you kind of smiled and grinned.

And for a moment, I felt that we had agreed on something. But at this moment, I think you are again repeating the same record that you had said before several times—that is very clearly stated—that you have problems with your feelings and that you have defenses that you are trying to control and that it is hard to talk about this, and you began as if nothing had happened but then it was like this idea and if you tell it to me several times, then I will not insist on asking you "what's the matter with you?" Let me tell you another reaction I have, and see whether this makes sense to you. I have a feeling that you are talking like the staff talks to you, as if you were imitating, reproducing how and what they tell you, at least as you remember it.

PATIENT: So it's really not what I feel.

You know I pick up things about myself from what other people say and how they see me, so its hard for me to . . . you know . . . really see how I feel about myself with all that's going on with me. I really rely on what other people say about me. That affects me.

[Exploring the patient's object-representations, the interviewer asks him about his therapist.]

THERAPIST: What is he like? Can you describe him? I know him a little bit but I don't know him very well. Since you have been with him so long, maybe you can tell me a little bit more. What how would you say he is like?

PATIENT: He's a really great man. I think he is. But er I'm scared to death of him. And er . . . I feel like there are times when he could just sit down and just play with my head and force me to let out these emotions that I guard so much, and there are times like this that I tend to get enraged at him. And rage is something I really can't deal with because when I get angry I feel powerful. I feel very destructive. And I don't know how to control that. I have a lot of rage towards a lot of people in this world and . . .

THERAPIST: You know something . . . ?

PATIENT: I'm sidetracking.

THERAPIST: How did you do that?

PATIENT: I don't know. I just . . .

THERAPIST.   How did you sidetrack just now? I was going to comment on the same thing . . . so . . .

    [His identify diffusion becomes evident.]

THERAPIST: You know . . . er, let me just elaborate a little on what you were beginning to say. I asked about Dr. _____ and you ended up talking about yourself.

PATIENT: You know, he's there to help me see what's going on with me and guide me through things, my difficulties.

    [The Patient could not acknowledge that he saw himself as interchangeable with Dr. ____.]

The interviewer, having observed numerous examples of the six variables in the interview, can sort out his or her observations and match them to the corresponding level of personality organization. Below is a summary of the several incarnations of the six components as they characteristically appear in the neurotic, borderline, and psychotic personality organizations.*

Neurotic Personality Organization

Cognition
- Subject presents a logical and thoughtful account. He has the capacity to focus, and at the same time, when asked, he is able to engage in elaborations that enhance and clarify his statement.
- Subject's account contains omissions of significant data although it remains logical. The account can be sparse, with minimal elaborations,

---

*These scales were formulated jointly with A. Carr, T. Cherbuliez, M. Selzer, L. Rockland, B. Fibel.

or full of excessive details. When omissions are pointed out to him, the subject acknowledges them and is able to elaborate relevantly.

Affect

- Affects are appropriate to content; there is a wide spectrum, and they are well modulated. The subject may spontaneously refer to the affective states of others (including the interviewer) as well as to his own.
- The range of affective responses is narrow and the capacity for modulation of affects limited; they are, however, manifested appropriately in terms of both content and interaction. The subject's description of affective states of third parties is more detailed than the description of his own or the interviewer's affects.

Self-Representation

- The subject refers to himself in all his complexity. He spontaneously discriminates between what is central within him and what is secondary. Contradictory or negative aspects of himself are recognized; he shows a capacity for and curiosity about further understanding.
- The subject is aware only of the broad outlines of who he is. The subject does not spontaneously acknowledge modifications to his self-concept. He is less curious about exploring more than what immediately meets his eye. However, he can acknowledge new aspects of himself when the interviewer points these out to him.

Object-Representation
(Refers to the internal representation of the relationship to others)
- People are described in a valid, distinct, and dynamic manner with discriminative features, both positive and negative, including physical and psychological traits.
- There is a tendency to place people into categories as well as to describe them with a few traits. The description does include positive and negative aspects but without much elaboration.

Ego- or Self-Reflectiveness

- The subject can easily reflect on his own behavior, verbalization, and affect, past as well as present. When his discourse presents a contradiction, he spontaneously reflects on it and its significance. When invited to, he easily puts himself in a position to reflect about an event in which he participated and to draw fresh conclusions about himself. He may also do so on his own.
- The subject does observe his own behavior, leaving occasional discrepancies between verbalizations and/or affect unnoticed. By and large he is successful at reflecting on issues if they are pointed out to him by the interviewer. The subject can miss subtle aspects of his motives and contributions.

Empathy

- The subject's capacity for empathy is demonstrated by his success at appreciating other people's positions, primarily the interviewer's, combining thematic and emotional components.
- The subject's capacity to empathize is preserved in most areas but shows limits in others. In those areas of limitation, the subject retains the capacity to register the interviewer's cognitive and affective themes but shows limits in his empathy to other people. When asked to discuss this further, he is able to integrate various aspects on his own.

Borderline Personality Organization

Cognition

- The subject's account can leave contradictions unresolved, but these contradictions may be acknowledged if the interviewer points them out. His descriptions give a two-dimensional flavor to his narration as he tends to describe issues in black-and-white. Thinking is dominated by a rigid, overly conventional, rehearsed quality.
- The subject's account is discontinuous and tangential. However, over time, with the interviewer's help the subject can make sense of his internal logic.

Affect

- Affect is appropriate to the content but inappropriate to the interaction. The subject may initially appear aloof and at other times overinvolved. He may oscillate abruptly in the expression of emotions. Affects tend to be demonstrated rather than described verbally.

Self-Representation

- The subject's relationship to himself is contradictory. One aspect of himself is presented as if it were the whole picture. (Sometimes he feels himself to be exclusively terrific and in other contexts exclusively horrible.) However, when the interviewer points out these polarities, the subject is able to present a more integrated view of himself.
- The patient tends to describe himself predominantly in terms of how others perceive him. The interviewer's efforts to elicit descriptions of his subjective experience are avoided or acknowledged without conviction. The interviewer's attempts to present a complete picture of the subject may be accepted fleetingly. The patient has little curiosity about himself, and his relation to himself is less crucial than the wary, vigilant attitude he holds toward others.

Object-Representation
(Refers to the internal representation of the relationship to others)

- Others are seen in terms of individual needs; their particular individual differences are not of immediate relevance. The other tends to be described in terms of function: "He helps me." "She works for me."
- Others are characteristically described in a generalized elemental and extreme way with no evidence of awareness of the contradiction, for example, "She is always nosy." "He is never kind to me."

Ego- or Self-Reflectiveness

- The subject observes his behavior only on request or along restricted lines. Further, once having observed, she appears to make no more use of the experience.

- The subject does not observe his own behavior. He can, however, agree or disagree with an observation presented to him by the interviewer but without any further elaboration.

Empathy

- Two qualities mark the subject's empathy: a sharp contrast between contexts where empathy is noticeable and those where it is absent, and abrupt shifts in empathy, which can follow the vicissitudes of the subject's own thinking or the interviewer's interventions. When asked to discuss further, he cannot integrate disparate aspects on his own; when confronted with them, the patient can recognize the incongruity.
- The subject's manifestations of empathy are quite limited and isolated from one another. His preexisting expectations of the interviewer may be mistaken for his showing empathy. The patient can recognize that the interviewer has a different point of view, yet he cannot accept it or integrate it.

Psychotic Personality Organization

Cognition

- The subject demonstrates idiosyncratic shifts in moving from concrete to abstract topics as well as concretizing abstractions and vice versa. The part may stand for the whole or the whole for the part. The subject may use pronouns other than "I" to refer to himself and pronouns other than "you" to refer to the interviewer.
- The subject's account contains illogical, idiosyncratic, and unfounded statements. Verbal production by the subject blends internal state with the external environment. Blocking, rigidity, and confusion of animate and inanimate may be apparent.
- There is no way to know whether or not the subject's responses are related to the interviewer or even to the present circumstances. The subject's account is a strange, disoriented word mixture. Although other people may be referred to, they are blended with any other context of the subject's utterances. There is no recognizable, constant relationship between the words the subject uses and the concept generally associated with the word.

Affect
- Affect is at times inappropriate to content and interaction. Affective states emerge unpredictably. There is pressure for action.
- Affect is disconnected from interaction and content, to the point of appearing incomprehensible. There may be a "flattening" of affects and rigidity.
- Intense, explosive affects involve gross motor systems, independent of current content and interaction.
- Affects are undifferentiated and diffused; their nature cannot be identified.

Self-Representation
- The subject's relationship to himself is initially difficult to determine because he can be quite constricted and guarded in his self-presentation. However, during the course of an interview, his guardedness is difficult to maintain, and what emerges is a rigid, constricted, and chaotic picture of the self. The subject is clearly attempting to hang onto himself for dear life. Although he can present himself as highly integrated, that representation is not objectively verifiable.
- The subject's experience of himself is elusive and shifting, often containing partial traits of others as if they belong to him. He may see himself as controlled by other people or machines. He may express a sense of loss of himself, but the acknowledgment will be fleeting, if it occurs at all. In an attempt to prevent further erosion of his sense of self, he may insist on defining himself by negation to an outside source ("That's *your* problem, doctor").
- The subject's representation of himself cannot be determined in any clear-cut way, as distinct from representations of objects or other persons.

Object-Representation
(Refers to the internal representation of the relationship to others)

- Objects are fused with each other; the symbolic and concrete are fused ("God and girls are the same"). Or self-representations are fused with God ("I didn't know you could be God and still be yourself").

3. Example: 6-year-old enacts his mother's gesture and appearance with a scarf on his head and by lifting tone of voice.

Humor

1. Definition: The play activity is perceived to be funny because of incongruity, exaggeration, or because it is amusingly unexpected. It is accompanied by or results in laughter.
2. Narrative Expressive: I'm taking some distance to see it from different perspectives, to master it while having fun.
3. Example: (A 7-year-old child, while laughing) "Boo! I scared you!"

Cluster Two

Intellectualization

1. Definition: The play activity deals with the emotional implications of the play in a neutral, actual, objective way.
2. Implicit Narrative: I am changing my experience into one of thoughts.
3. Example: "Here comes the fireman. He knows all about putting out fires." (Child goes into detail describing what the fireman knows about burning buildings.)

Rationalization

1. Definition: The child explains the play to the therapist using acceptable but false reasons.
2. Implicit Narrative: I will give myself a different reason to avoid worry.
3. Example: The child puts the family of dolls to sleep on the bed except for the baby, which she puts on the floor, stating that there is no more room on the bed.

Isolation

1. Definition: In the play activity, ideas are separated from their threatening affects; the result is often an apparent indifference.
2. Implicit Narrative. I am separating an idea from its associated feeling.

3. Example: A 9-year-old girl (with neutral affect) offers the therapist a piece of "spider-poison pie."

Doing and Undoing

1. Definition: The play activity is carried out and then reversed or neutralized. There is an underlying representation of equal opposing wishes. The cyclical quality of these play events may cause them to appear magical.
2. Implicit Narrative: I am placing it and then taking it away.
3. Example: The child gives the baby doll the bottle, then takes it away, and then gives it back, only to take it away again.

Negation

1. Definition: In the play activity, the child dismisses the value, meaning, or significance of the threatening feeling or behavior.
2. Implicit Narrative: I know it could be great, but I don't care.
3. Example: The therapist is winning the Monopoly game and is making a lot of money. The 9-year-old boy says he is about to win; he only needs to get the chance card, and then he will win.

Reaction-Formation

1. Definition: In the play activity, a warded-off idea and feeling are replaced by an ungenuine expression of its opposite. Reaction formation keeps the painful idea and affect in mind; only the value is reversed.
2. Implicit Narrative: I am putting forward one side of my experience rather than the other.
3. Example: Child is carefully and "lovingly" making a Playdough doll, making it very "beautiful." Then she yanks it off the table, disconnecting the head from the body.

Repression

1. Definition: In the play activity, the child successfully plays out a theme of which he is unaware.
2. Implicit Narrative: I am holding it in. I'm not looking, I'm not seeing, and I'm not aware of it.

3. Example: A child with a sick parent plays out going to the doctor and getting a healthy report.

Projection

1. Definition: In the play activity, qualities, feelings, wishes, thoughts, or roles which the child refuses to acknowledge are attributed to another person or toy.
2. Implicit Narrative: I am putting this outside of me into someone/ something else.
3. Example: A 7-year-old plays that Godzilla will destroy all the people one by one, whereas the child with the good superheroes will protect the people.

Introjection

1. Definition: In the play activity, one character transposes objects and their inherent qualities from the outside to inside his own self. The emphasis is on being the recipient in the interaction.
2. Implicit Narrative: We experience the traits of another inside ourselves. (I am swallowing, taking this into myself.)
3. Example: (Child) "The small guy swallows a special pill the big guy gives him. Now he can be strong too."

Regression

1. Definition: In the play activity, the child or her characters revert to modes of activity and expression typical of a younger child.
2. Implicit Narrative: I am turning backward in time.
3. Example: Child pretends she is being a younger child. A 7-year-old looks for an object to be a blankie or sucks on a doll's bottle while talking baby talk, or a school-aged child wants to make a big mess.

Somatization

1. Definition: In the play activity, the child or one of the characters is preoccupied with physical symptoms.
2. Implicit Narrative: My body is speaking for me.

3. Example: In the play activity, the little boy doll stays home from school because he has a headache.

Turning Aggression Against the Self

1. Definition: In the play activity, an unacceptable impulse is redirected by the child or one of the play characters against himself.
2. Implicit Narrative: I'm hitting myself.
3. Example: (Child) "Batman just shot his own weapon directly at himself."

Avoidance

1. Definition: In the play activity, the feared object or character is turned away from (maybe fleetingly or momentarily). The child has construed the feared object or person as a threat to her functioning and withdraws from the situation in a phobic way.
2. Implicit Narrative: If I turn away from the danger, I won't even notice it.
3. Example: The child walks away from the witch puppet, negating its presence, with no hint of interaction.
4. Example: The child plays turning her back to the therapist.

CLUSTER THREE

Denial

1. Definition: A mode of defense that consists of refusing to recognize the reality of a traumatic experience, a painful affect, or a sector of the external world.
2. Implicit Narrative: I am shutting off, closing myself off from that (painful) experience. I make believe it didn't happen or it doesn't exist
3. Example: The girl doll is about to be eaten by the dinosaurs and goes on peacefully eating her ice cream.

Splitting

1. Definition: An active process of keeping apart attributions concerning the self or the other, with lack of concern and denial of contradictions. The split-off attribute is so threatening that it is not recognized as be-

longing to part of the self or as part of the other person (i.e., the lack of synthesis of contradictory self and object images in idealization and devaluation).

2. Implicit Narrative: Two contradictory aspects of "me" and the other "person" are separate and disconnected from each other.

3. Example: The Raggedy Ann doll is so very good at the beginning of the session and is played with; then she (the doll) is so bad, she is abruptly thrown away. Each part of the play activity may be accompanied by intense polarized affect.

Projective Identification

1. Definition: Externalization of bad-aggressive aspects of the self or object images into objects that are experienced as dangerous. Fear of retaliation makes the subject defend himself by keeping others under control to prevent them from attacking.

2. Implicit Narrative: The object (or experience) is outside me. "I" am actively holding it at arm's length so that it does not return into me.

3. Example: Robin and Batman are on guard against the bad guys; they have to be ready for action, or their "evilness" can pop up at any moment by surprise and attack.

Primitive Idealization

1. Definition: The person or object is valued above all others because of a characteristic(s) that cannot be duplicated. The unattainable attribute(s) cast a magical, powerful spell, giving power and authority to the other(s).

2. Implicit Narrative: The object is perfect, pure, kind, and powerful. I am not much in comparison. The object is "high" above; I am "below."

3. Example: (Child, referring to one of the play characters) "Sam is a great player, and he is so smart. He can never be beaten."

Primitive Devaluation

1. Definition: The child devalues the other(s) completely. She is rejected as disgusting and abhorrent, dismissed as having no importance, and may appear sinister or threatening. At this level, the devaluation is

complete and focuses on one characteristic (or set of characteristics) that causes the other to be unacceptable, with no redeeming features.

2. Implicit Narrative: You are no good.

3. Example: (The child playing teacher, to her student, played by the therapist) "You are stupid; you are too dumb to answer the questions. See how I do it!" (Proceeds to draw scribbles on the blackboard.) "I'll show you!"

Omnipotent Control

1. Definition: The child attempts to control the external world by being all-powerful and coercive, with the expectation of being treated in a special way.

2. Implicit Narrative: I must keep everyone under my control.

3. Example: (Child playing with his mother and therapist) "I'm the boss of the universe. You guys stand up here, don't talk, I'm the superhero, I'm the one to talk, shut up, you are out."

Identification with the Aggressor

1. Definition: Identification with the "bad object" who intrudes and aggresses upon others. By playing the strong person, the child quells her anxiety about being weak and vulnerable.

2. Implicit Narrative: I am big and strong and can do with them as I please.

3. Example: The child plays at being a strong soldier who injures the villagers.

CLUSTER FOUR

Dedifferentiation

1. Definition: Several different items lose their separate identities and become homogeneous. Order is removed from an organization, rendering it chaotic.

2. Implicit Narrative: Things are mixed together regardless of their original specific function.

3. Example: The contents of the toy shelves are dumped into a disorganized pile, and the child leaves.

Constriction

1. Definition: An extremely persistent, preservative, rigid repetition of cognitive thoughts, affect, and behavior. All three must be present. It involves a significant narrowing of the self or the child's perception of the other.
2. Implicit Narrative: Everything must stay in one area, limited to the same story, same beginning and ending.
3. Example: The child jumps from the table to the floor in a monotonous, repetitive way, with a frozen grin.

De-animation

1. Definition: Rendering an animate object lifeless.
2. Implicit Narrative: It is still, not doing anything.
3. Example: The child brushes the therapist aside as though she were a piece of furniture.

Dispersal

1. Definition: Dangerous aspects of the self and the other are broken into fragments and scattered. (Note: The object may be disparate pieces, such as Legos—the whole object need not be formed concretely in order to be scattered.)
2. Implicit Narrative: Aspects of the self/other must be broken into pieces and spread around so as to make it not dangerous anymore.
3. Example: Lego pieces are taken out of the container and scattered all over the playroom.

Dismantling

1. Definition: The process of reducing the person or toy to disconnected segments.
2. Implicit Narrative: It is disconnected, as parts of the body, or as themes unrelated to each other.

3. Example: The doll's feet, legs, and arms are dismembered with scissors; the hair of the doll is cut off and thrown around the room.

Autistic Encapsulation

1. Definition: Throughout play, the child conveys a process of insulating herself from her surroundings and her therapist. Play is an all-encompassing, protective barrier.
2. Implicit Narrative: It is walled around me and inside my mind.
3. Example: The child hides under the table and remains unresponsive in the session.
4. Example: The child turns around and around, becomes mute, turns her back to the therapist's communications, and does not respond to sound or touch. She resorts to self-stimulating activity (e.g., rocking, humming).

Fusion

1. Definition: The concomitant blurring of boundaries in the area of differentiation between self and non-self into a state of oneness.
2. Implicit Narrative: Discrete things get lost in a boundlessness with everything.
3. Example: The therapist observes the child putting together the Playdough queen doll and the Playdough witch doll figures, and now they are mixed together.

Freezing

1. Definition: A process of halting the functioning of the person for the purpose of survival.
2. Implicit Narrative: To control my terror I make everything stop and stand still.
3. Example: The child pretends to be a statue or becomes motionless.

Hypocondriasis

1. Definition: A dangerous feeling or impulse is experienced as residing within a particular body organ, a body organ that can destroy the individual. It represents a transformation of reproach for others into a body pain.

2. Implicit Narrative: The negative intentions are taken in again and feels bad.
3. Example: The potion is made, and the doll child has to drink it; she wants to get rid of it, but nobody can make her tummyache go away.

Reversal of Affect

1. Definition: The appropriate affect is replaced by the opposite, often a bizarre and inappropriate substitution.
2. Implicit Narrative: The affective experience is so terrifying that it needs to be silenced by excitement and laughter.
3. Example: Laughter for fear. The clue to the presence of a transformed affect is often in the incongruous, or incongruent, experience of the therapist.
4. Example: The therapist listens to a frightening story told by the child, which is accompanied by excited giggling.

All these mechanisms can be assessed in the interactions with the adolescent during the interview, as well as in play in the case of younger children (P. Kernberg et al. 1998) because these defense mechanisms are implicit narrative expressions used for purposes of dealing with extreme anxiety or depression. During a PAI, a 15-year-old was asked what she had been told about the interview. She responded that she was supposed to see the greatest doctor, and she had indeed heard that the interviewer was a very good psychiatrist. Yet when the interviewer did not join her in her complaints about her parents, the patient shifted to saying, "You are here only asking dumb questions. You are stupid." Her inability to reconcile that statement with the fact that, minutes earlier, she had been absolutely convinced that the interviewer was "the best doctor" indicated the appearance of splitting, primitive idealization, and devaluation.

Similarly, in one child's play narrative, the little girl doll invited the adult dolls for a nice lunch and was behaving beautifully when suddenly she served a poisoned soup that would kill all the guests. This abrupt transformation is a typical expression of splitting mechanisms (P. Kernberg et al. 1998). The play context is a forum for the spontaneous expression of personality traits. If we believe that children have personalities and that they can have personality disorders, the play interview will yield valuable Axis II information.

ASSESSING REALITY TESTING

The assessment of reality testing will differentiate between borderline personality organization, in which the reality testing can be lost but regained, and psychotic personality organization, where reality testing is lost.

Reality testing is maintained if there are no hallucinations or delusions; if the capacity to differentiate self from non-self is intact, along with the capacity to empathize with the clinician's intentions and purposes (e.g., his observations on inappropriate peculiar characteristics of the patient behavior); and if the patient's explanation about behavior in the session is congruent with the reality testing of the therapist. Otherwise, reality testing is lost. For example: The patient is looking away from the therapist, the muscles in her cheek are twitching, and she looks as if she is omitting something. The therapist discusses her observation of the patient's face. The patient acknowledges and accepts the therapist's observation and adds that, indeed, she was feeling nervous because she did not want to tell the therapist that she had been drinking the day before.

The capacity to differentiate animate surroundings from inanimate is another criterion of reality testing. Children who can enter fantasy play and then leave to resume everyday interactions exhibit reality testing, as when a girl is playing at being the queen on a throne surrounded by her servant dolls, the therapist says, "Time is up," she stops her play, goes to her mother seated in the waiting room, and asks, "Are we going to McDonalds now?"

ASSESSING STRUCTURAL CHARACTERISTICS:
PSYCHOLOGICAL TESTING

The application of current theoretical concepts to traditional psychological testing has yielded diagnostically valuable characteristics on projective tests. Psychological testing, integrated with a detailed diagnostic interview, reveals the presence and the severity of features that underlie personality disorders.

The specific projective tests that appear the most useful include the Rorschach Test, the Thematic Apperception Test (and its analogues), and the Sentence Completion Test. Each of these tests presents children with a task that is indirectly more effective in revealing personality characteristics than direct questioning about the child's thoughts, feelings, and experiences. The Rorschach Test, in particular, is uniquely powerful in eliciting pathological functioning that can be empirically compared with nonpatient populations starting at age 5 and that can specifically address cognitive, affective, interpersonal, and ideational aspects of the child's functioning. The material that follows is based on clinical work and also on initial research findings of a study of children with narcissistic personality disorders (Bardenstein 1998).

Test Behavior

The child's test behavior provides information that informs the description of his personality development. Important data about personality functioning can be gleaned from the child's reactions to the examiner's attempts to manage his behavior and the countertransference the child's behavior engenders, as well as from his manner of dealing with the test.

It is reasonable to assume that all children are anxious when they begin testing. Thus, the initial meeting with the child provides one index of her level of anxiety and her means for dealing with it. Some children easily and eagerly leave their parents and go from the waiting room to the examination area. They include those who are motivated to impress the examiner and their parents and/or to confirm their own high, perhaps inflated, self-regard; those who try to do well so that others will not think there is anything wrong with them; and those who are more trusting and understand that they may get something from the evaluation, such as help in school or a better self-understanding that will help them and their parents.

For other children, the best they can hope for is to avoid destruction, attack, humiliation, or abandonment for poor (or good) performance. These children include those who are more likely to show a borderline level of organization and occasionally a psychotic loss of distance with test material, indicating lapse of reality testing. The anxiety in these children is palpable.

A 6-year-old girl with significant learning disabilities, a developmental language disorder, and an attention deficit disorder would sometimes duck under the table during the administration of cognitive tests. While viewing Rorschach Card VI (which commonly can have phallic and aggressive associations), she revealed that the unusual hand movements she made at times were designed to scare the examiner. She was afraid of the toy helicopter she saw because "shooting can sometimes come out of the antennas." Although she seemed to realize it was only "pretend shooting," her confusion of animate and inanimate features signaled her thought difficulties. Her hiding under the desk because she was afraid that the examiner would kill her was readily managed by turning it into a hide-and-seek game; she easily laughed, became playful, and returned to the testing. This provided her with an enduring means for mastering the anger she felt and projected onto the examiner whenever she was presented with difficult test material. Whenever she felt frightened, she would disappear, hide-and-seek would ensue, and she would then continuing working.

Some inpatient children require a different approach. For example, one elementary school–aged girl was upset by the Rorschach. On Card II she said, "This is a girl, no, it's not. Blood, blood. It's a jelly fish." Card III was "A lobster. Know what makes it? Blood. Is this blood?" Card IV, which can have phallic overtones, was met with "Get that one away from me, too." She ran to get a stethoscope in another part of the room and, in a break with reality, asked, "Are you Dr. L?" (her therapist) and then ran out of the office. She returned with "her" nurse, continued testing while the nurse sat off to the side, and said Card V was a "bat," an excellent, popular response. Thus, with additional support, she was able to recover and have restored reality testing.

Older and more intact children, such as those with narcissistic features, may comment about the test or the examiner ("This is easy," "Anybody can do it," "How long have you been doing this?"). Children with oedipal-level concerns may often ask about how they are doing and wonder if they compare favorably to other children. Others may act out their competitiveness and try to take over by completing instructions or beginning to respond before the examiner has finished his part. The need to perform well is also seen in some children's attempt to cheat by looking behind the screen as the examiner sets up the WISC-III (Wechsler Intelligence Scale for Children, third edition) Object Assembly items.

COGNITIVE TESTS

On structured intelligence tests, schizophrenic patients show intrusions of primary process material and thought-disordered responses. Borderline patients, both adults (Bern 1983, Gartner et al. 1989) and children (Leichtman and Shapiro 1980a, Leichtman 1988), can also show moderately severe thought-disordered responses. It can be assumed that, in most outpatient cases, the greater the intrusion on the structured tests, the more serious the psychopathology. Incorrect responses often provide the vehicle for the expression of intrusive conflictual concern (Berg 1983), and the child's asides and behaviors provide considerable material.

A child's personality organization can impact both the content and the type of his responses to the structured intellectual tests.

- A 10-year-old depressed girl, who did not provide any human responses on the Rorschach Test and instead saw only "crushed" nonhuman figures on each card, misheard the WISC-III Vocabulary word "fable" as "feeble" and defined it as "a newborn calf can't walk well, that's feeble."
- A 10-year-old narcissistic boy with many somatic complaints said one WISC-R Picture Arrangement sequence portrayed a "kid hitting his father with a bench, and the people in the back are cheering." This same youngster defined "hazardous" as "dangerous, you're in danger to everyone, including yourself."
- A depressed, narcissistic 14-year-old boy illustrating his grandiosity defined "prevent" as "stop you from doing something, like pulling a switch to blow up the world".
- A seven-year-old depressed, masochistic boy, whose misbehavior seemed designed to elicit punitive, attacking reactions from others (as if to ensure that he would not be happy), defined "nail" as "something that protects your finger".
- A 12-year-old narcissistic, borderline boy, whose first Rorschach response was "two people trying to pull an ant apart" and who was struggling with his own sense of splitting fragmentation, defined "nail" as "something that holds something else together".

Neither of the latter two children could simply say, "A nail is something that you hit with a hammer," a more common response.

Intrusions are not restricted to Verbal IQ subtests. A 9-year-old boy spontaneously commented on the WISC-R Block Design subtest, "Say, I never knew there would be blood in the sky" as he reproduced a pattern with red and white blocks. This same youngster commented that the first WISC-R Object Assembly items, which required that he put puzzle-like pieces together to make a girl, "looks weird." When asked why, he said, "Because the arms and legs are chopped off, and the head is flying around in circles." The castration concern reflected in this response was also evident on the Sentence Repetition Test, a receptive language task that merely requires the child to repeat the sentence that has been read to him. This boy, when read a sentence about a father "giving his boy a beating," would not repeat it because he said, "I don't know what that is." The use of denial was so blatant and pervasive in this case that it is small wonder that the child's learning was compromised and that he had been referred for testing for school-related reasons.

The information conveyed in the examples just cited does not, in itself, provide the basis for a diagnosis. These cases do illustrate, however, how cognition can be compromised by emotional factors and how cognitive tests provide additional data that increase one's confidence in the validity and reliability of findings from the projective tests. They also indicate, for some children, the pervasive impact of the PD that consistently affects so much of their functioning.

PROJECTIVE TESTS

Personality testing by use of projective tests, such as Rorschach Test, Thematic Apperception Test (TAT), and Figure Drawings, examines such areas as level of reality testing, presence or absence of a thought disorder, affective experience and expression, representations of self and other, capacity to relate to others, defensive style, capacity for sublimation, developmental level and drive organization, and reactivity to situational demands.

This section will focus on some of the information obtainable from the Rorschach Test. It is assumed that the child will approach this task as she would any other, so that her usual coping mechanisms are expected to be displayed. Standard Rorschach administration procedures can be used by 5 years of age, along with basic scoring procedures and response interpretation (Leichtman 1988). By this age, children realize that the Rorschach card is a representation and not a picture and that they must justify their response for the examiner to be able to see it; fantastic responses become the exception.

The Rorschach can be viewed as a perceptual/cognitive task that examines how a person structures and organizes ambiguity (Erdberg 1990). The formal scoring procedures are an attempt to quantify and to analyze how a person does this. They evaluate the number of responses and the part of the card (whole, large detail, small detail). Responses are also accessed for consensual accuracy (form level), color and shading of the cards, and the tendency to see human and/or animal movement. These elements are stable in adults; those that are not reflect situational variables and can be expected to fluctuate over time (Weiner 1986). Children show less test/retest stability than do adults, but J. Exner (1995) reports that the stability increases with age. This pattern is similar to longitudinal descriptions of repeated intelligence testing (Kagan and Moss 1962). Structural information reflects a person's problem-solving style, and inferences from it are generally more accurate than inferences from the thematic content of the responses (Weiner 1986).

REALITY TESTING

The form level—the "goodness of fit" of a response to configurations of the ink blot—is taken as an index of reality testing and the capacity of the child to view his world in a conventional fashion. Can the examiner see what the child sees after the child explains his response? Is his response reflective of what is seen by other children of the same age?

This variable is extraordinarily stable. For example, repeated testing finds the same form level (Exner 1995). Thus, low form level by an elementary school–aged child indicates impaired reality testing, and the perceptual inaccuracy or vagueness of his response should not be attributed merely to his being a child. This finding is consistent with the finding that loose associations do not occur in normal children over 7 years of age (Caplan and Sherman 1990). In effect, the establishment of concrete operational reasoning (Inhelder and Piaget 1958) seems to bring with it an accurate view of one's world; deviations from that conventional, realistic view are pathological.

THOUGHT DISORDER

There are several indices of thought disorder that can be derived from the Rorschach Test (Rappaport et al. 1968) and that reflect different degrees of severity (Exner 1993). They relate to verbalizations, combinations of ink blot areas, and logical inferences. The juxtaposition of examples of adult responses (Exner 1995) with responses from children illustrate that the impaired perception and reasoning is apparent at any age.

Deviant Verbalizations may be neologisms ("a woman with a *disretheal* air about her" [Exner 1993, p. 166]) or redundancies ("a pair of *two* birds"

[Exner 1995, p. 166]). They may include inappropriate phrases ("Some kind of bug but I've never seen one like it; *neither has anyone else for that matter*" [Exner 1995, p. 167]) or circumstantial material ("It looks like a map *I can tell because I've traveled a lot. A map that represents darkness and light*" [Exner 1995, p. 167]).

Inappropriate combinations create unrealistic relationships between perceived objects and attribute inappropriate activities to them. In varying degrees of severity, they represent greater or lesser violations of the boundaries and identity of the object (Blatt and Ritzler 1974). *Incongruous combinations* condense details or images and merge them into a single object ("a butterfly with his hands out" [Exner 1993, p. 168]). A 9-year-old outpatient boy responded to Card I, "Bat with his hands up."

Fabulized combinations always include two or more objects in the blot for which an impossible relationship is described ("two ants fighting over a baseball bat" [Exner 1993, p. 168]). A 12-year-old inpatient girl responded to Card VIII, "Looks like two animals up a hill. A head. Looks like two animals going up somebody's head. I mean his hat." A 6-year-old outpatient described Card X as "two pink worms shaking hands."

J. Exner (1993) also includes transparencies here ("Here is a man, and you can see his heart pumping" [p. 168]). A 7-year old outpatient described Card VII as "the inside of a toad. Because it's brown; because toads are brown."

Contaminations are the most bizarre responses to the Rorschach Test; when they occur, they are usually found in schizophrenic patients. They are fusions of two or more percepts into a single response in a particular, discrete part of the blot. The result is a violation of each individual percept in the creation of the fused image. It is as if the identity of the percept is destroyed ("It must be a bird dog 'cause it's got the body like a dog and nose of a bird" [Exner 1993, p. 168]). A 12-year-old inpatient girl said of Card III, "Looks like two animal people. Looks like apes, people, animals, both, they're animal people." A 7-year-old outpatient responded to Card VIII, "I got a good idea of what this could be. It looks like a fish bird to me. This looks like the bird part, and this looks like the fish part." One 10-year-old inpatient was so upset by his impaired thinking and his failed attempt to recover that he experienced further deterioration in his reasoning and overall functioning, which also reflected attitudes about himself at that moment. In response to Card VI, he said "An ant lion. I mean a lion monster. Erase all that! [*He seems agitated and very upset.*] All I see is a piece of shit lying on something."

Several types of responses reflect disordered thinking and indicate poor logic and inferences. *Autistic logic* is Exner's (1993) term for a form of loose thinking in which the person's reasoning is based on the size, position of the blot, or the number of objects included in the response ("This green must be lettuce *because it is next to the rabbit*" [Exner 1993, p. 169]). In *confabulation*, the subject generalizes a whole response on the basis of just a small part of the blot. The whole blot is included even though it does not fit with the response, but the subject does not seem to realize that or attempts to justify the answer ("a claw, a lobster" [Exner, 1993 p. 171]). A 10-year-old female inpatient responded to Card I with "A lamb because of the ear." Finally, in *fabulization*, the response is affectively elaborated in a manner not justified by the blot itself. A 10-year-old female outpatient described Card III as "an angry woman."

Developmental Analysis of Projective Testing

There are many response elements to the Rorschach Test that indicate the same psychological processes in children and adults but must be interpreted according to developmental level. Consider responses involving the color on the blot. The use of color reflects how one deals with emotions and responds to emotional experiences. Very young children might just name the color. When older children do so ("It's blood, it's red"), very poor management of emotions is indicated. Responses in which the person's percept is determined primarily by color (C) with the form (F) of the object as secondary, signify less restraint and depth in expressing emotions, which are more shallow ("It's a leaf because of the color," scored as CF). Alternatively, greater emotional control and depth of emotions are represented by responses in which the form of the percept and color are both used, but the form is the primary determining characteristic ("a butterfly because it's shaped like a butterfly and it's red" scored as FC). As expected, nonpatient adults generally provide at least twice as many FC as CF responses. The opposite is the case with children, who normally give more CF than FC responses. A child who gives more FC than CF answers, replicating a normal adult pattern, tends to be emotionally inhibited. Adults may find such children to be pleasing, even mature, but the children do not do well with peers.

A similar analysis can be made with human and animal movement responses on the Rorschach Test. It is possible to see a human on the

Rorschach without attributing movement to it, or the figure may be seen as active (jumping, giving "high fives," fighting) or passive (sleeping). Animal movement (scored as FM) is illustrated by responses such as "a beaver climbing a mountain"; human movement response ("two people cooking," scored as M) is related to many positive features about the use of one's inner resources, such as intellect, the capacity to delay immediate responses and thereby be more reflective and creative, and the use of imagination. Its absence is a cause of concern and, if the form level of the M response is poor (M-), it can indicate poor interpersonal relations and is more likely to be seen in schizophrenics (Exner and Weiner 1995). M responses, more frequent among adults than in children, increase during childhood; animal movement decreases in frequency with age and is taken to imply more unorganized ideation than M. In adults, impulsivity is expected when FM appears more frequently than M in a test record.

Schwartz and Eagle (1986) suggest that it is not until children are 12 years of age that the frequency of M and FM equalizes. Exner (1995) reports norms that show similar trends; for preadolescents, FM is greater than M. Campo (1988) reports that there is a greater likelihood of a variety of serious disorders when M is greater than FM in prepubertal children. She asserts that it is maladaptive for the child to be using an adult defensive style, which can result in an inflexibility in dealing with change and a premature establishment of character structure.

PROJECTIVE MATERIAL AND PERSONALITY ORGANIZATION

The Rorschach Test and other projective tests measure personality processes; they are not designed to directly assess *DSM-IV* diagnostic categories, and one should not look to them for single, specific signs to make an Axis I or Axis II diagnosis in children or adults. It is possible, however, to delineate multiple complex characteristics that describe the personality disorders and to find elements of Rorschach behavior that correspond to them, as has been done with diagnosis of such conditions as schizophrenia, depression, and conduct disorders (Weiner 1986). It is the evidence accumulated across the many Rorschach responses of a subject, together with the person's performance on the other projective tests and the structured cognitive tests, that allows for confident statements about personality organization.

Cognitive Functioning: Flexibility and Resistance

Children with PDs have difficulty accurately perceiving details of both the external world and their internal states. Their skewed and rigidly sustained world views maintain their beliefs, ward off anxiety, and keep them from feeling overwhelmed. Signs of impaired reality testing, rigid mind sets, and an overly simplified black-and-white interpretive approach are common features of the projective material. In the Exner Comprehensive System for the Rorschach (1986), the relevant structural variables include significantly high Lambda (oversimplification of stimuli and avoidance of nuance and complexity), high X- or Xu percent (distorted or idiosyncratic perception), and significantly discrepant active-to-passive movement ratio (rigid, inflexible mind set). The content reflects this constriction and lacks richness and depth. Often, one category, such as monsters and other malevolent creatures, absorbs the child's attention. Verbal material on the Rorschach, Apperception, and Sentence Completion Tests is often terse and superficial; the child attempts to deliver safe, concrete, and nonrevealing information about thoughts and feelings.

Affect

Emotional development is stunted in personality-disordered children because their limited repertoire of coping with others deprives them of growth-promoting emotional exchanges. They prefer to control and contain emotional experiences because of the potentially destabilizing effect of their rigid and therefore fragile resources and defenses. Emotional constriction is readily seen on the projective material in the avoidance of any mention of intense emotion (minimal color content), the narrow range of emotional experiences depicted, the limited number of responses to color-dominated cards (an unwillingness to process affect), and the atypically pseudo-mature inhibition of spontaneous affective experience indicated in the higher ratio of form-dominated responses over color-dominated responses. '

Aggression, anger, and alienation are apparent in both the structural features of the Rorschach Test (elevated space responses) and the content (themes of fighting, pulling away, engulfing, and eating). In the study of narcissistic children, orally aggressive creatures, such as dragons, or figures equipped with weapons, horns, stingers, or poison surfaced in the majority of the children's Rorschach protocols. Sadistic, pleasurable exploitation of others, a feature characterizing narcissistic and antisocial personalities, appeared as well; often, weaker objects were at the mercy of larger, malevolent figures. The affective attitude of a child is revealed as to whether he identifies with the victim or the victimizer. Rather than expressing distress, concern, or discomfort with such images, the narcissistic and/or antisocial child is amused by such predicaments.

Affective constriction is evident in the nature of activity between objects on the Rorschach Test. If the interaction is not aggressive, it is parallel at best, with an absence of involvement and reciprocity.

INTERPERSONAL FUNCTIONING— SELF- AND OBJECT-REPRESENTATION

The history of affective constriction and absence of mutuality also emerges in the cluster of Rorschach features called the Coping Deficit Index (CDI). A positive CDI characterizes people who are inept or who are interpersonally chaotic or ineffective. They lack the emotional resources and flexibility to manage the demands of interpersonal relationships. Character-disordered children rely on rigid, limited coping styles that interfere with the development of intimate, supportive, and reciprocal relationships. Because reality in general is distorted and misinterpreted, the perception of others and their motives is equally subject to distortion. On the Rorschach Test, quasi-human figures (e.g., ghosts, fairies) and human details dominate wholly human figures. The inability to accurately read others' and one's own internal state affects empathy and understanding. Nuances are missing, and a black-and-white view of others often polarizes people into good and bad caricatures. Children with character disorders often project onto others their own unacceptable flaws, aggression, and neediness. On the Rorschach, such children also score positively on the Hypervigilance Index (HVI). HVI is characterized by a constant state of preparedness against potential external malevolence. Personal space is zealously guarded, and others' motives are automatically suspect. This theme arises in the content of projective story and sentence completion material as well.

SELF-PERCEPTION: IDENTITY

Because the child's interpersonal experience, emotional adjustment, and cognitive functioning are all organized to secure the maladaptive personality structure, the experience of self is also affected. Without accurate interpretation of experiences and a broad emotional palette to register and to respond to others, the child unknowingly deprives himself of an accurate, reality-based, and balanced self-image.

An impoverished self-image results, with a constant sense of inadequacy in comparison to others, and it appears in projective material in several ways. Structurally, the Rorschach Egocentricity Index—a measure of self-focus—is significantly lower than expected. Morbid content, in which objects are ruined, damaged, or disintegrating, is common as a self-experience. The increased ratio of part human and quasi-human percepts to whole human percepts on the Rorschach Test is another common feature, indicating that the self-representation is likely based on fantasy and is immature for the age level.

Some children with personality disorders, specifically the antisocial and narcissistic disorders, attempt to buttress their weak senses of self by inflating their attributes and externalizing all negative qualities onto others. In a Rorschach study of narcissistic children, the number of reflections (mirror images or reflections of objects in water) was, indeed, higher than in the nonpatient population. Reflections on the Rorschach empirically correlated with an inflated sense of self and a concomitant need to preserve and protect that inflated sense by denying flaws or deficits. Paradoxically, the Egocentricity Index was still depressed, even though the number of reflections contributed to the score. The narcissistic children's senses of self colored the content as well. Grandiose, embellished, and idealized images occurred in the majority of the subjects; damaged, idealized figures were also common, such as "Batman with holes in his wings."

The Sentence Completion Test also provides rich information about the sense of self. Many items require self-reflection, a difficult task for children with atrophied self-images. Certain items, such as "The worst thing I ever did was . . ." and "The biggest mistake I ever made was . . ." are particularly difficult because self-criticism is a common deficit in these children. An antisocial child replied that the worst thing he ever did was to kick an opponent in the head during a soccer match. He added that the boy deserved it because "he was in the wrong place at the wrong time." A narcissistic child replied, "The biggest mistake I ever made was to come here and talk to stupid psychologists!" These children prefer to give conventional, superficial, or concrete responses either defensively or because they do not know themselves well enough to articulate anything meaningful.

The images of self and other, not unexpectedly, are equally superficial in tasks involving storytelling. On the Thematic Apperception Test and the Children's Apperception Test, stories can reveal pathological interpersonal paradigms consistent with the child's PD. One narcissistic patient described figures typically seen as a daughter and her mother as a mother with her sister, as if to displace her mother and demote her to equal status. Power relationships, control of goods, and control of malevolent forces are frequent themes, reflecting the impoverished self.

Human figure drawings can provide corroborative material with respect to cognitive maturity assessed both empirically and via clinical interpretation. The insubstantial quality of the self and object world can be conveyed by figures lacking distinctive features, such as gender-related details or figures done factory-style. One patient drew a sequence of heads, followed by bodies and limbs, then facial features, to depict his family. His drawing had an assembly line quality to it. Inadequate figures with lavish embellishments, such as jewelry or elaborate decorations, suggest the attempt to compensate for an inferior sense of self.

In summary, cognitive, affective, self, and interpersonal aspects of the personality-disordered child appear in projective material in distinctive ways. Signs of inflexibility; inaccuracy of perception; compromised emotional functioning; interpersonal deficits; and a weak, inadequate sense of self appear in both the structure and content of the Rorschach and in tests involving drawing, storytelling, and responding to incomplete sentences. These observations should be considered preliminary findings to be progressively evaluated as further research continues. The clinical and research material is consistent with predictions based on the theoretical understanding of this population and provide guidelines for assessing possibly personality-disordered children.

PART III
THE NEUROTIC
PERSONALITY ORGANIZATION

III.1

Introduction

The personality disorders that comprise the neurotic cluster are the mildest in the diagnostic spectrum; as such, they allow for the highest level of personality functioning. Before examining their particulars, we must address two conceptual issues associated with the neurotic cluster and its application to children and adolescents.

The first is the problem of differentiating what constitutes symptom from what constitutes personality. The literature on anxiety disorders, for example, looks at anxiety as an isolated symptom, serving as its own target for observation and intervention. The notion that a specific anxiety may be embedded in an overall maladaptive organization of related personality traits is rarely considered. The absence of a comprehensive system for personality evaluation to determine if a given symptom is truly an isolated or situational phenomenon or whether it exists in a matrix that supports the behavior in an ongoing, inflexible manner is a significant weakness in approaching the research, diagnosis, and treatment of childhood disorders.

The second issue is the lack of clarity between what can be developmentally expected and what represents an atypical variant.

Patients identified as having one of the four neurotic personality disorders—Hysterical, Obsessive-Compulsive, Avoidant, and Self-Defeating (formerly 'Masochistic')—share a similar characterological organization. It is distinguished by an integrated sense of self, including both positive and negative features, and a capacity to view others in a similarly realistic way; some capacity to tolerate anxiety and control impulsivity; an integrated, albeit harsh, superego or conscience; and the ability to establish nonsuperficial relationships with others, recognizing each person's separateness and uniqueness.

Stone (1993) observes that all four disorders also share another feature: inhibition in the assertion of socially acceptable impulses. Such impulses may include sexual, aggressive, and irritable feelings that are reluctantly, if at all, expressed in interpersonal situations. Stone characterizes these disorders of inhibition as "ego dystonic": They cause subjective suffering despite the symptoms' integration into the personality structure. The neurotic patient is likely to internalize blame for his or her difficulties, beyond any basis in reality, and to own the symptoms—in contrast to the borderline, narcissistic, and antisocial personality-disordered patients, who externalize blame.

The neurotic level personality-disordered patient is more likely to engage in and to respond better to treatment.

III.2

Hysterical (and Histrionic) Personality Disorders

DEFINITION

There is no hysterical personality category as such in the *DSM-IV* system, but we conceive it to be the counterpart in the neurotic organization to the histrionic personality (borderline organization), which *DSM-IV* does describe, as "a pervasive pattern of excessive emotionality and attention seeking. This pattern begins by early adulthood, and is present in a variety of contexts" (p. 655), and it is signaled by at least five of the following criteria.

- Patient is uncomfortable in situations in which he is not the center of attention.
- Patient's interaction with others is often characterized by inappropriate sexually seductive or provocative behavior.
- Patient displays rapidly shifting and shallow expression of emotions.
- Patient consistently uses physical appearance to draw attention to self.
- Patient speaks in excessively impressionistic style lacking in detail.
- Patient self-dramatizes, behaves theatrically and exaggerates expression of emotion.
- Patient is suggestible and easily influenced by others or circumstances.
- Patient considers relationships to be more intimate than they actually are.

The intensity of these traits and the degree of identity integration and self- and object-development (Horowitz 1977) define a continuum corresponding to the severity of the PD. The hysterical personality manifests a milder form in the neurotic personality organization, whereas the histrionic personality represents the most extreme form and belongs alongside borderline, narcissistic, and antisocial personalities in the borderline organization (O. Kernberg 1992, Akhtar 1992).

The incidence of hysterical and histrionic personality disorders in childhood and adolescence is unknown. References to both categories are scarce in the childhood literature (Metcalf 1991).

JEANNIE—AN ADOLESCENT WITH HYSTERICAL PERSONALITY DISORDER

Jeannie, a 15-year-old, was referred to one of the authors for treatment. At the beginning, both Jeannie and her parents talked about her chronic unhappiness with herself, her tension and her anger, and negative and hypercritical attitudes toward herself and others, including a deep resentment of her brother who "could do everything better than she."

Overall, Jeannie was quite a good student. She excelled in dramatics, foreign languages, and sports. The second of four siblings of college-educated parents, Jeannie had longed for her real father, whom she lost in her early childhood through divorce. Although her mother remarried after a few years, she deeply resented her stepfather and the children born during the second marriage, a girl and a boy, five and seven years her junior.

OVERVIEW OF DEVELOPMENT

There were no medical complications in pregnancy and delivery. At the time of her birth, her parents were in intense marital distress, characterized by violently angry scenes. Her mother described Jeannie as a healthy, vigorous, easy baby who made her needs known by her distinct crying.

Developmental landmarks were within normal limits. When she began to speak, she spoke clearly, and she learned to read at an early age, teaching herself phonics.

Jeannie went to preschool and elementary school with no apparent problems. As she entered adolescence, she became more distant from her mother, and her relationship with peers deteriorated. She was competitive with her peers and siblings and frequently complained of being shortchanged by her parents in relation to her male siblings. Although generally she seemed to control her affects, she had intense temper tantrums if something did not go her way.

As a teenager, she was stern, conventional, and prudish. Although at times she liked to exhibit herself by sunbathing in a bikini on the terrace of the roof of the building or by wearing tight clothes, she would express outrage if the boys made comments about her looks. She had a boyfriend, whom she "just liked as a friend." She liked to be held by him but discouraged other expressions of affection. She complained that he only wanted to "neck" with her and was concerned that her reputation might be spoiled if she went steady with him.

She described her two sets of parents in a rather generalized, nonspecific manner; the most blurred figure in her description was the father. She had chronic difficulties with her family and felt she didn't get along with either her mother and stepfather or her father and stepmother. Lately she felt she had no close friends.

It was striking to observe that in spite of Jeannie's attractive appearance and well-developed secondary feminine characteristics, she behaved in a sexless, frozen manner. She was controlled, talking with a certain deliberateness that served the purpose of suppressing many intermediary thoughts. In addition, she selected words that were global and not specifically descriptive.

The process material that follows is from psychoanalytic sessions that occurred after Jeannie had been coming for intensive insight-oriented psychoanalytic psychotherapy. It reveals many of the characteristic styles of hysterical personality disorder. Jeannie's comments highlight her sense of frustration and disappointment in her mother and explain her resultant demandingness.

The contributing factors of Jeannie's sense of maternal deprivation need to be specified. In Jeannie's case, maternal deprivation meant intermittent emotional unavailability because of her mother's stress in her first marriage and divorce. In addition, her mother showed a preference for Jeannie's half-siblings. Furthermore, there was a special kind of deprivation in that her mother tended to relate to her child in a narcissistic manner. Jeannie's mother expected her daughter to suffer from the same psychosomatic illness she did. Because her mother anticipated many of Jeannie's concerns, Jeannie became quite dependent on her mother to find out how she felt about things.

The tendency to somatization:

After a tense visit with her father and stepmother, Jeannie proceeded to report unpleasant details in a calm manner that surprised the therapist in view of the content. *"When I got back, my stomach started to act up. I also had blotches and pimples all over the place, which hardly ever happens—stomach, heartburn a monumental case of it. I got my whole face broken out and I ate like crazy. I also have tension in my head, vague headaches, awful, pain in my left eye, throbbing. It got better and then it got worse. I also have a tension headache when I am here [in session], and it goes away when I leave."*

Sexual inhibition and guilt:

The patient expressed intense inhibitions and guilt over sexual strivings, both toward the boyfriend and in the therapy situation, and dealt with them by means of repression and a dissociative experience during the session.

Referring to their vacation, she said, *"A couple of things happened that I did not want to think about. Tom and I, we did a little more experimenting in our sexual life, which I regret. I don't want to think about it."* Jeannie said that her boyfriend was happy about it, but she was regretful and upset; she talked about her petting with her boyfriend, her enjoyment, and her fear of loss of control. Then Jeannie began to describe a dream.

It was weird, strange. There were other people. You and I were in a library, and I was waiting for you to come in. You were in another room with another patient. I was poking around in the office. In the middle of the room there was a big blue book—it was a physician's desk reference. I looked up stomach medication. I wanted to look for . . . Instead I found it was a book about diseases. We were trying to classify what my disease was. It was very strange. You turned the pages, you read all the symptoms—excessive eating, not sleeping—that always sounds like you. There was a light brown chair. We were looking at my disease. There were awful symptoms that described me.

She could see that her sexual experience with her boyfriend was linked to her fear of punishment as expressed in her fear of the terrible disease in the dream.

A Dissociative State:

After she described her difficulty in petting with her boyfriend, Jeannie commented:

Weird, I didn't know how to think about the sessions. Last time I was here, it felt as if I was in a trance. I felt as if I had been listening to myself in a trance; I came out of it confused, embarrassed, not sure what you were going to say about it. I felt spacey, not all there—scared. While I was talking a wave of strong feelings came over me; I felt confused. I wonder, was it like a sensation? It was very sudden, a big wave just hit me very strong. I felt like laughing and crying—mostly in my head, I guess. Like my thinking about something which is very wide and blank—it is peculiar and hard to describe. It was when [I described the dream where] you were looking through this book to find out what disease I had, again, I felt peculiar, giddy, faint, like crying. I was in a trance, yet I kept talking; when I was finished with the dream I kept talking. I wonder if I made the whole thing up . . .

The therapist asked her whether it was similar to the experience she had had with Tom that she could not describe. She said it was similar; she did not feel good at all.

I felt seasick. I also regret it at the same time. Now he has some control over me that he didn't have before. I have a large grudge against men in general. I felt like fainting, too. It would prevent me from losing control, not doing anything else. For a while he necked, petted, but he felt that he wanted to be working for my climax. If I told him my feelings, he would have more power over me than I think he should. I didn't like to give him the idea that he matters more to me than he does. It would make him feel good. He should not think he was so wonderful for me. He should think it was mostly my doing. I feel that I am not going to solve it, what does it matter, anyhow.

I started to have a headache now, like my head would fall apart when I leave here. I am going to regret bringing this up.

Jeannie's cognitive style can be seen in a fragment of her description of her subjective experiences in a session a few weeks later:

I am pretty tense all the time. I never seem to get the grasp of the idea of a conversation. [This in spite of the fact that she was an outstanding student.] *I can be more relaxed with some people, but I want to make sure that people will like me. Sometimes it is worse with friends. It is more important that I appear favorable to them. (Sigh.) Usually it results in my feeling false most of the time. I think sometimes friends like you for what you really are; the person I seem to be is nonexistent.*

Everything I do has fizzled away, and at school I am not doing much of anything anymore. My oldest brother, he has kept his interest through the years, and by now he is a good saxophone player.

I have it all there, but I can't seem to do anything with it; I have all the qualities. I know, but I don't read enough. I don't think enough. I could be a good musician. I haven't done anything with my talents. It is almost as if you didn't have them.

In treatment she began to connect with her sense of her depression, diffuseness about feeling that something was missing in her—the deep roots of her perception of being a girl, an incomplete being, and her envy of men.

TINA: A CHILD WITH
HYSTERICAL PERSONALITY DISORDER

The case of Tina, a 6-year-old child, has some striking similarities to the hysterical personality described in Jeannie's case, in spite of Tina's much younger age.

When Tina's parents came to see the therapist, they felt she needed treatment because of her extremely negative reaction to the birth of her younger brother, two years her junior. She had found his presence overwhelming; she had teased and provoked him. When she first saw her baby brother being diapered, she shouted, "What is that?" from the doorway. Her overall functioning had deteriorated. She now asked for things to be done for her, to be given to her, and yet no matter how much her parents did for her, she always felt that it was not enough.

She didn't get along with other children. She would initiate contact, but after a few minutes, she would manage to antagonize all her peers. This situation had happened with eight girls in her class. Nobody wanted to sit next to her. The teacher, in fact, had to persuade somebody to sit next to her, and the child who sat next to her eventually hated her.

There was a driven quality to Tina. Initially she could be charming with other children, but then she let them know that she could do better than they could, that they were stupid. Often she said, "That's not right, stupid," to any child who was doing something contrary to her wishes. She found herself compelled to needle other children. She refused to share her toys. She wanted very badly to have friends, but children rejected her. The only friend she had was a boy at school who could stand her provocativeness because he didn't seem to care. She was extremely hostile with her brother. She stirred him up, and when he brought his friends home, she goaded them to antagonize him: "See that little boy? Don't let him in. Let's punish him." Although her behavior with her parents was better when her brother was not around, she still was quite unpleasant. This behavior had grown worse.

She read very well at school, but her desk was an absolute mess, and she was forever losing her pencils. She had no sense of responsibility. Although at times she showed some creativeness, she did not apply herself and was described in the class as a drifter. She was always losing her library books, her milk money, and her notebook. Earlier, in nursery school, Tina was described by her teachers as wonderful, creative, although somehow shy with other children. Toward the end of nursery school, however, she began to be more withdrawn, as if something was bothering her.

Tina's parents reported repeatedly during the consultation session that she was never satisfied. Due to her oral demandingness, even on her birthday her mood was completely spoiled because she worried about not receiving enough or the same as the rest. She ate voraciously. She piled up her plate even though there was already a lot on it.

Developmentally, the parents described a normal pregnancy and delivery. Tina weighed seven pounds at birth. She was a wonderful baby—responsive and active. She was breast-fed for two months but did not gain enough. During her first year of life, she was kept on a schedule of feedings every four hours.

Language development was advanced, and at 2 years of age Tina was able to talk in rather long sentences and to carry on advanced conversations.

During the diagnostic evaluation, Tina drew herself consistently larger than her parents and especially her brother. In fact, in the drawings, she took two large pages to draw herself at a size of approximately 20 inches tall. In contrast, her brother was meekly drawn as a fragmentary stick figure without arms and hands, two inches tall.

Both her mother and father worked. When the therapist met Tina for the first time, she was of average size, with big blue eyes and honey-colored hair. She moved and dressed rather unattractively. Her shoulders were humped. There was a quality of suffering about her that reminded the therapist of a miniature Madonna. Often she came theatrically dragging a long multicolored scarf on the floor. Then, when she entered the playroom, she put it on; she looked like a grand dame wearing her stole. She was indeed unhappy about practically all aspects of her life.

On one occasion well toward the end of the first year of treatment, Tina painted a flower. She then painted another flower, and progressively this flower turned into a messy, brownish surface. She did the same with a third flower. She then proceeded to paint her hands and her elbows. At this point, the therapist told her that maybe at times she felt good about herself—like a pretty flower—but maybe then she thought she had done something that made her feel all messy, like this brownish stuff she was smearing all over herself.

Tina had consistently omitted any talk about masturbatory activity. At this point, the therapist commented on this omission, saying that maybe there is something that makes her feel so dirty and bad, such as her playing with her genitals, rubbing herself, or touching herself. She looked at the therapist with surprise and said, "No, I never do it. My brother does it, pulls his penis hard, and he hurts it. He does it all the time, even in concert." She added, "I really like to watch it." The therapist pointed out that Tina never talked to the therapist about it—maybe she felt it was something very bad to talk about or do. She replied that nobody does it at school. "When I go to the bathroom, I do it, and it hurts a lot, you know, it really hurts. I am the only one at school who does it." Tina and the therapist talked about how difficult it must be, and how if she did not know that other boys or girls also did it, she must feel even worse.

At this point, she proceeded to paint her face like a clown while looking at herself in a portable mirror that the therapist had in the office. She painted her mouth big in red and continued to paint brown all over her face, expressing her sense of messiness about masturbation.

She began to read a book on how babies are made. She looked with considerable interest at the drawings of flowers and puppies, but when human examples came up, she closed the book rather hurriedly and said she knew all about that because she had seen a TV show. When she saw the rooster on top of the hen, she said, "They can't do it like that," with a sense of disbelief. Then she commented that she didn't know how it was with humans because she had not seen it. On the TV show there was a real woman. They had an adopted child. She is not adopted. She expressed the universal fantasy of the fear of the destructive penis upon penetration, hence, her disavowal of sexual intercourse.

Her particular links to father (seductive) and to mother (dependent) were illustrated in a nightly ritual. Tina had a special way of saying goodnight to her parents. With her father, she kissed him on the mouth, and with her mother, she complained of her aches and pains. Tina referred to it by saying she liked to talk with mommy and that she had nothing to say to daddy. As she became more autonomous, she relinquished these rituals and became more involved with peers and a boyfriend. She was able to work through her anxieties about envy of boys, her oedipal rivalry with the parent of the same sex, and her conflicts and guilt about masturbation.

PAT—AN EIGHT-YEAR-OLD WITH
HISTRIONIC PERSONALITY AND NARCISSISTIC TRAITS

Pat was referred at the age of 8 years, 3 months, for an evaluation to assess her emotional and cognitive functioning, using the WISC-III; the Achenbach Child Behavior Checklist; and the Rorschach, Draw-a-Person, Sentence Completion, and Thematic Apperception Tests. Psychological testing yields an in-depth view of a child whose histrionic personality with narcissistic traits puts her at the more severe end of the hysterical spectrum.

Pat is currently in treatment with a therapist who describes her as a challenging patient who is not forthcoming with her feelings and not easily engaged. Her parents and stepmother are concerned about Pat's pseudo-maturity: She tries to act grown up and wants to do adult things. She feels entitled to control and manipulate others' play, activities, and conversation; she can be intrusive and overly preoccupied with what her mother wears. With respect to her divorced mother's relationship with a man, Pat is jealous and hostile; she wants to have a boyfriend, too. Her lack of consideration for others is another source of concern, as is her seeming indifference to being punished for misbehavior: She neither learns from nor shows remorse for her mistakes. Finally, the patient continues to suck her thumb and demand her "bop," a piece of her mother's torn robe, when she needs to soothe herself.

At first, Pat was immediately friendly and talkative, showing the examiner the contents of her backpack and chatting in a high-pitched voice. She announced that she did not like her name and wanted to be called Mary or Karen. Whenever she was asked about any problems or difficulties she might be having, she complained about others in her life.

She asserted that Peter, her mother's boyfriend, "strangled me in Hawaii" because he did not permit her to get a Kleenex, and she showed equal resentment that he had sent her mother flowers on her birthday but that she (the patient) did not get any. Pat added that she had heard about a girl having sex with her stepfather, and she expressed jealousy of her mother's having sex with Peter; she said she wanted to have a boyfriend and to have sex, too. When asked what she understood "having sex" to mean, she replied that it was "too sick" to talk about. She asserted that things would be better if she could be a teenager and drive her own car; also, she complained that Peter was too mean and too rough. While talking, the patient put her feet against the chair, sucked her thumb, and held the "bop" that she had removed from the backpack.

Pat was cooperative during the cognitive parts of the testing but clearly became increasingly irritated with the more ambiguous, projective testing that called for expression of personal thoughts and feelings. As she seemingly felt more threatened by the material, she became openly devaluing of the examiner and engaged in more oppositional behavior. She began to throw a soft football around during one projective test; she continued to do so even after she was asked to stop, until a clock was knocked over, whereupon she expressed no concern about her actions.

At the third and last session, Pat was hostile and demanded to be present at the feedback session that was being arranged. Simultaneously, she asserted she did not want to come back and see the examiner again. When her behavior was reflected back to her—specifically, her difficulty in addressing questions about how she feels about herself—her response was to become further enraged and tight-lipped. Nonetheless, the patient conveyed significant aspects of her personality style, ways of coping, deficits, and concerns.

Mother, father, and stepmother independently completed the Achenbach CBCL. The three profiles were in striking agreement with respect to borderline significant pathology in the Delinquent Behavior Index. Lying, cheating, lack of guilt, and preoccupation with sex were among the items endorsed.

mate with animate in a single object indicated a disregard for conventional boundaries and a comfort with bizarre fantasy. The cognitive confusion continues in the following response: "It could be Ohio . . . no, never mind . . . the whole world . . . United States . . . is Florida the United States? But it isn't Florida, so you can cross it out."

Pat is able to sustain a most intact presentation in the presence of structured intelligence testing. She is alert to convention and can respond appropriately until pressed by unacceptable demand. She senses when she may be under threat (of being, e.g., disciplined, criticized, left out of the sphere of attention, thwarted in getting her needs met). She is likely to become angrily oppositional and negative in such situations, further compromising her ability to assess herself and others accurately.

It is clear from the content of the Rorschach Test as well as the other projective test and the actual responses to the testing situation that the patient becomes more flustered and disorganized when having to deal with her affects. Her needs become her reality. When asked, for example, what made an inkblot look like ice cream, she angrily answered, "because I'm hungry for ice cream!" The testing itself became increasingly disturbing to the patient, who devalued the Rorschach as "boring" and expressed her anticipation of being done with it so she would not have to come back, and she could then have some fun.

Pat's rage and devaluation barely disguise how vulnerable, incompetent, and ineffectual she feels at a level beneath her awareness. She struggles with a mixture of sadness and emptiness, which she tries to fill by extracting and demanding what she needs from others, yet she is wary of being dependent (viz., her desire to be an adult who needs nothing from her parents). Images of food are associated with her dependency needs: In one response, she saw a huge dish of ice cream overflowing its container, and in another a man with "a big bladder [sic] . . . he's got all these things for the babies to suck out of." On the Sentence Completion, she said, *When I eat,* "I want more."

Pat wants badly to be the one controlling the goods; otherwise, she feels intolerable envy and resentment, as her attitude toward her mother's relationship with Peter confirms. In one poignant and revealing response, she described seeing "an animal with a lot of antennas, and he's inside a huge cage, and there are flames and smoke like a fire in there." The theme of antennas and their connection to vigilance is juxtaposed with a character deeply endangered but trapped beyond others' help; it captures Pat's fragile, tormented self that must be hidden and guarded at all costs. Many of the patient's intellectual resources are deployed in this endeavor.

Her self-perception is characterized by extremes. Her self-esteem is markedly poor; this patient ruminates on her faults. One image, "A bug dressed up in a tuxedo," depicts a lowly creature in elegant trappings—yet her last Rorschach response, describing a woman with a bra in royal robes, shaking pompoms, is exhibitionistic and grandiose, defensively narcissistic in quality.

Responses on the Sentence Completion Test echo both the grandiose defenses and the sense of impairment that produces Pat's conflict and distress (which are then externalized): She expresses the desire to be a model—but she depicts her father as critical of her wherewithal to do so.

She blocks on such items as *When I think about my body* ("I don't know . . . I don't . . . I don't think about it"); and *When I look in the mirror* ("when I see myself . . . I . . . don't know . . . I don't do anything"); *My hands* ("are fat . . . my fingers are fat . . . I don't want them").

Any invitation to be self-critical is fiercely warded off by devaluing others: *My biggest mistake was* "I talk to psychologists . . . it's stupid . . . Why can't I be like everyone else? The pills aren't doing anything. They're stupid and they waste my time." *The worst thing about me is* "I have to take pills and go to psychologists." The fantasy of being all powerful and rich is used to enhance the sense of self. Pat chooses not to admire anybody when invited to do so: *I want to be like* "like have magical powers . . . I could make people fly and make people disappear"; *What I want more than anything* "is to be rich and have slaves."

The interpersonal implications are profound. Pat remains emotionally constricted, difficult to get close to, relentlessly vigilant, and feeling entitled to special treatment. Her neediness is so pressing that she bends or disregards the rules or misinterprets them altogether, requiring external control and vigilance because she cannot tolerate or cannot experience self-critical feelings of guilt and remorse. If she fails to impress someone, she dislikes him or her completely (*I don't like* "people who don't like me"), as her derogatory view of Peter suggests. Pat's inability to admire others was evident in her hesitation to respond to the prompt: *The other kids in school are.* She explained that if she said they were funny, the evaluator might assume that she is not funny. Complimenting others would detract from how she is perceived.

A synthesis of the foregoing findings suggests that this patient has a chronic, maladaptive set of personality traits and cognitive deficits congruent with histrionic and narcissistic personality disorder. Diagnostically, she fulfills the criteria for both, as marked by a relentless need to secure the self against others' criticism or demands, a constant need to be given to and envy of others who have what she lacks, an inability to reflect critically about herself, externalization of blame and responsibility onto others, and a desire to be admired and catered to by others. In pursuit of these needs, she feels entitled to violate rules of conduct without remorse and to ignore boundaries.

The fragility of Pat's sense of self is inferred by the degree to which she attempts to exert control, as well as her regressed self-soothing. Through controlling, devaluing, and distancing others, she tries to maintain the fantasy of a perfect, mistreated child who deserves unquestioned fulfillment of her needs. The patient's cognitive resources are diverted into seeing things as she wants to perceive them to the degree that reality becomes distorted and misconstrued. She is, accordingly, vulnerable to disordered, peculiar thinking that remains fixed.

Because close relationships are fraught with difficulty (i.e., triggering envy, the withholding of goods, potential criticism and demands, emotional reactions), Pat is wary of engaging others in a mutual fashion. She is left with a chronic sense of emptiness and the nagging conviction beneath her awareness that she is inferior. The very defenses that protect her preclude the possibility of a reality-based, integrated sense of who she and others are; her capacity for empathy, remorse, and reciprocal love are currently arrested. Symptoms of depression, irritability, and anxiety are likely to surface with time.

COMPARATIVE PERSPECTIVES
AND DIFFERENTIAL DIAGNOSIS

The range of the childhood hysterical personality, from mild to severe, conforms with the general classification of high-level and low-level character organizations described by O. Kernberg (1976), as well as, more specifically, with the high-level and low-level hysteric described by B. R. Easser and S. R. Lesser (1965) and the "good hysteric" and the "bad hysteric" described by E. Zetzel (1968).

The hysterical neurotic personality, Zetzel's "good hysteric," implies a well-integrated but severe and punitive superego, a well-integrated ego identity, a stable self-concept, and a stable representational world. Excessive defense operations against unconscious conflicts center on repression. The characteristic coping and defense behaviors are largely of an inhibitory or phobic nature or are reaction formations against repressed instinctual needs. There is very little or no evidence of direct sexual or aggressive instinctual infiltration into the defensive personality traits. The ego at this level is somewhat constricted by its excessive use of neurotic defense mechanisms, but the patient's overall social adaptation is not seriously impaired.

The hysterical personality has fairly deep, stable object relations and is capable of experiencing guilt, mourning, and a wide variety of affective responses. The sexual and/or aggressive drive derivatives are partially inhibited. However, the infantile genital phase and oedipal conflicts are clearly predominant; there is no pathological condensation of genital sexual strivings with pregenital (oral and anal) aggressive impulses (latter predominating), as is typical in the borderline organization group of personality disorders (Abraham 1920, Easser and Lesser 1965).

Characteristic traits surface frequently enough to provide evidence for clinical descriptive or face validity. Differences along gender lines (Blacker and Tupin 1991) emerge in children and adolescents.

GENDER DIFFERENCES

Boys
Boys are pseudo-masculine, hyper-masculine, macho, with superficial affects, and subject to denying feelings. Their exhibitionism is expressed through risk-taking behavior. Sexuality is used to gratify dependency needs and is characterized by promiscuity and premature ejaculation.

Girls
Girls are pseudo-feminine, seemingly incompetent, subtly passive, indirectly manipulative, and emotionally overreactive. Their exhibitionism is expressed through seductive behavior, provocative dress, and surprise at the resulting response. Sexuality is used to control the partner and to coerce dependency characterized by frigidity.

PATTERNS IN HYSTERICAL PERSONALITY

M. J. Horowitz (1977) identifies long-, medium-, and short-order patterns common to the adult hysterical personality, representing durations of weeks, hours, and minutes respectively, during which they surface.

Long-order patterns (perceived in terms of weeks). Interpersonal relations are repetitive, impulsive, and stereotyped, often characterized by victim-aggressor, child-parent, and rescue-rape interaction. The hysterical personality creates cardboard fantasies, conceives of caricature-like roles, and leads a drifting but possible dramatic life with an existential sense that reality is not really real. The self is frequently experienced as not in control and not responsible.

Medium-order patterns (perceived in terms of hours). The hysterical personality shows attention-seeking behavior, which may include demands for attention; the use of charm, vivacity, and displays of sex appeal; childlikeness; passivity; or infirmity. There are fluid changes in mood and in motion, with excitability and an episodic flooding with feeling. Inconsistency of attitudes and suggestibility are also present.

Short-order patterns (perceived in terms of minutes). The information-processing style involves global deployment of attention and unclear, inhibited, or incomplete statements of ideas and feelings, possibly with a lack of details or clear labels in communication. Nonverbal communication is not further translated into words or conscious meanings; there are only partial or unidirectional associational lines with a short-circuiting of the completion of problematic thoughts.

It is important to distinguish the hysterical personality from the phenomenon of conversion in order to approach treatment appropriately. L. Rangell (1959) defines *conversion* as an expression of forbidden wishes in symbolic form or via body language; it may also serve as a way of escaping life-threatening stress at almost any age or stage of development and in almost any pathological personality configuration. The sicker patients are, in terms of their level of object relations, their use of primitive mechanisms of defense, their early fixations, and their problems in the integration and maturity of the ego's synthetic functions, the more blatant and infantile their conversion symptoms will be.

The relationship between symptomatic hysteria and the hysterical personality type is unclear. The reports in the literature of overt hysteria have not been related to personality style. L. Robbins (1966), for example, shows that girls diagnosed with hysteria during childhood were only slightly more susceptible than nonhysteric girls to falling ill with hysteria in adult life. None of the boys with hysteria in childhood had such symptoms when they grew up. In this study, however, there is no reference to the Axis II diagnosis of hysterical personality as such.

DEVELOPMENTAL PSYCHOPATHOLOGY

We first turn our attention to the role of endowment in the formation of personality, specifically of hysterical traits; then we will address the influences of early interaction with family, caregivers, and the cultural surroundings. A. Korner (1967) points out the difficulty of establishing clear connections between neonatal and later behavior. This difficulty is not surprising because developmental factors proceed toward an ever-increasing complexity and differentiation, which, along with a constantly changing behavioral context, obscure continuities. Nevertheless, Korner's description of individual differences suggests some predisposing links to hysterical traits.

The experience of self as not in control, the demands for attention, the fluid change in mood and in motion, the excitability, the episodic flooding with feeling, the inconsistency of attitudes, and the global deployment of attention with the lack of details or clear labels in communication—R. Gardner's (1968) levelers of childhood—are all quite possibly related to Korner's endowment factors.

INDIVIDUAL DIFFERENCES IN RESPONSES TO EXTERNAL STIMULI

Babies differ in their perceptual styles and types of defenses. Some respond to auditory stimulation with a large repertoire of reactions while others respond with only single or global bodily responses. Singular or global versus multiple responses to external stimuli may be, as Korner has suggested, a sensorimotor antecedent of later "leveling perceptual modes" (Gardner et al. 1968) and of repressive tendencies. Gardner and his colleagues found that "levelers," in contrast to "sharpeners," show more difficulty in perceiving similar stimuli as distinct in various sensory modalities; this incapacity negatively affects learning tasks and recall. In later observations of children between ages 9 and 13, Gardner and colleagues found that perceptual style is quite constant over time and shows sex differences; girls are more characteristically levelers whereas boys are more characteristically sharpeners. (Note the implicit correlation here with the *DSM-IV* criterion concerning excessively impressionistic speech lacking in detail.)

The infant's response to multiple and competing stimuli may be related to a predisposition to hysterical personality. During ophthalmological examinations, some babies suck more strenuously when the eye examination begins; others stop completely. This variable may relate to later tendencies of the hysterical child toward motor discharge or to displacement behavior aimed at tension reduction. It may foreshadow the need for warding-off mechanisms or a propensity to flood the ego apparatuses in the face of massive stimulation. (These considerations resonate with *DSM-IV*'s collective criteria of self-dramatization, theatricality, and exaggerated expression of emotion.)

Distinctness of state. Babies are more expressive and defined in their states of pleasure and displeasure. This characteristic makes it possible for the mother to read and respond to the cues given by the infant with more precision. It is interesting to speculate that if the mother does not attend to these cues, the child may have to exaggerate them to communicate them and avoid a sense of frustration and deprivation. The tendency to dramatize could have roots here.

Mode reliance. Observations of neonates show that there are individual differences in the quality of mouthing: Some clearly prefer sucking or tonguing, and others prefer chewing; some infants are droolers, others are spitters, and still others hardly ever spit. In E. H. Erickson's (1959) terms, the infant's mouthing may be primarily incorporative, retentive, eliminative, or intrusive in character. Whether early preferential-mode reliance reflects a lasting and distinctive drive quality, which then finds expression in later development, arises as a salient question. Is early mode reliance transferred to later psychosexual states, and does mode fixation thus influence personality development? For example, is the eliminative mode related to the tendency toward dissociation in the hysterical character? Or is the incorporative mode related to the orality, demandingness, and penis envy of these patients?

Another aspect of mode reliance is self-consistency, the capacity to respond to a stimulus in a predictable manner. (Hypothetically, this variable may be crucial to the ease with which a mother can learn to understand her infant's needs.) Unpredictability may be a function of fluctuations in the strength of internal stimuli impinging on behavior. The hysterical personality displays sudden, abrupt changes in behavior and moods in the form of shifting affects, and these may well be rooted, at least in part, in this particular factor of self-consistency (viz., the rapid shifting and shallow expression of emotions cited by *DSM-IV*).

Peak excitement. The level at which the infant's response to stimuli peaks is also a factor of heuristic interest (Brazelton 1973). The infant may go from a low level of response to stimuli to high-level reactions of excitement, such as screaming. This high-pitched excitement can end in an insulating crying state from which the infant is unable to be quieted or soothed. A predisposition to intensive affective reactions is indeed evocative of the histrionics and affective outbursts of the hysterical personality.

The Relation of Early Modes to Cognitive Controls and Defenses

A. Korner (1967) postulated continuity between early modes of processing stimuli and later cognitive styles or controls as proposed by Gardner and colleagues (1968); Gardner, in turn, linked cognitive controls to defenses. Indeed, Gardner and his collaborators have found a definite correlation between cognitive control and type of defenses. Much of their evidence, like that found by M. J. Horowitz (1977), suggests that the cognitive-control principles are structures antecedent to the formation of the defenses. The study of variations in the way neonates deal with external and internal body stimuli may thus clarify the antecedents to the formation of defenses.

In Gardner's study (1968), middle-class Midwestern children participated in various cross-sectional and longitudinal investigations, including clinical interviews, psychological testing, and some experimental testing related to cognitive structures. Gardner and his colleagues found that the characteristics of ego organization seemed as clearly defined in the clinical test performance of the younger children studied (average age of 9.6) as in the performance of the older children (average age of 13.4). These findings suggest that even in normal children, defense mechanisms are already employed in a more crystallized way than assumed earlier.

The study found, further, that those children who were levelers—that is, who lagged behind in the capacity for discrimination of similar stimuli—showed an inaccuracy of reality testing, demonstrating relatively high degrees of sporadic disruption of control in the clinical testing situation. The findings also suggest that there is a difference in the distinguishable capacity of boys and girls to articulate experience, with boys being more articulate (Gardner et al. 1968). This capacity is linked to relatively limited repression and relatively high scores on the WISC verbal factor. Children with low verbal scores, more often girls than boys, responded more quickly and willingly to the inkblots and gave responses to partial smaller areas of the inkblot; they also used repression to a greater degree. The link between field articulation (intelligibility, distinctive) is inverse to the level of repression and corresponds with findings of other authors, as does the superiority of boys over girls in the cognitive-control tasks specifically requiring articulation under relatively difficult conditions.*

In addition, Gardner and colleagues found that girls showed less explorative behavior; they seemed to be more placid and less open to new experience, less projective, and less verbally skilled. Similar descriptions are included in Horowitz's discussion of the cognitive styles of the hysterical personality in adulthood, suggesting a continuity into adulthood of these patterns.

Clearly, various studies of individual differences in infancy and latency suggest that specific endowment factors may contribute to the formation of the hysterical personality structure.

CULTURAL, PSYCHODYNAMIC, AND INTERPERSONAL FACTORS

Cultural practices may foster hysterical symptomatology and character. They may be codetermined by gender stereotypes affecting relationships between the sexes and tolerance or prohibition of sexuality (O. Kernberg 1992) or by gender role attributions (e.g., whereby girls are expected to be submissive, dependent, or shy).

A. Metcalf (1977) has best systematized the variety of psychodynamic factors depending upon the child. A selection of his factors follows:

Mother-child attachment bond. The insatiable attention-seeking of the hysteric may originate in part from the "insecure" experience, in which there is a partially frustrated attachment behavior. The partial frustration has the paradoxical effect of increasing the behavior rather than extinguishing it. Caregiver inconsistency enhances the effect on the child as seen in the case of the mothers of insecurely attached children of the ambivalent-resistant type (Main 1993).

---

*This general pattern of behavior was also more apparent in Catholic than in Protestant children. D. Beres (1969) stresses that character pathology needs to be assessed within the context of culture, and the value of doing so is amply illustrated here. Indeed, those children who were more open, uninhibited, and cooperative and who employed generalized repression to a lesser degree were more often Protestant than Catholic. This has interesting implications in that in predominantly Catholic countries or in Catholic subcultures, the incidence of classical forms of hysterical neurosis is higher than in Protestant countries and subcultures.

Reactions to physical illness. W. Abse (1974) points out that the parents of a hysterical child are often neglectful when the child is healthy and then remorsefully attentive when he is sick or distressed. Gratification and guidance can only or can best be supplied by the parent. Although such parents encourage the child to look and interact with others, they covertly signal that they are the most reliable source of support, and that guidance and gratification can only or can best be supplied by them.

Suppression of anger and assertiveness. M. Sperling (1973) describes how certain mothers do not permit expression of anger, assertiveness, or anxiety in their children but encourage dependency and passivity instead.

Inappropriate sexualization of the parent-child relationship. If parents develop an eroticized and physically infantilizing relation to a child, they may restrict other explorations in the environment.

A. Metcalf (1977) was the first to propose the existence of a spectrum of hysterical personality types from the "hysterically inclined child," a variation of normal personality. Children with hysterical personalities initially come across as outgoing, engaging, and charming and then become markedly irritating, intrusive, impulsive, and more selfish, according to Metcalf. Superficially dramatic and intense, they modulate their responses in keeping with their impact on the adult, whom they use as a need-satisfying agent (colloquially, a "sugar daddy"). One of the most impressive traits of such children is their uncanny sensitivity to the moods and unexpressed thoughts of the adults with whom they have relationships.

SEXUAL BEHAVIOR

The sexuality of the hysterical personality in childhood is deceptive. The overly feminine or seductive traits are only superficially sexual; they really express identification with the seductive parent(s) and represent a means of retrieving or maintaining love or the acting out of hostile manipulations. The child can easily become overly excited and prone to temper outbursts.

The hysterical personality met in early childhood turns to the father as a caregiver, usually due to frustration and/or deprivation in her relationship to her mother. In the context of marital conflict between the parents, this connection to the father can become an exaggerated enactment of the normal oedipal one. Both father and mother may encourage a sexualized relationship between father and daughter, facilitating her submissiveness and demandingness.

LEARNING SKILLS

Most children with hysterical personality disorders suffer some deficit in their cognitive development with the inevitable limitations in learning tasks. Their absorption in eroticized relationships with adults leaves them with limited capacity for the mastery of learning (Metcalf 1977); moreover, their global repression of data and their egocentric thinking inhibit their absorption of information in depth (Gardner and Moriarty 1968).

MECHANISMS OF DEFENSE

The milder hysterical child uses normal to neurotic defenses (i.e., identification with the mother, repression of the awareness of the sexual element in her own behavior, reaction formation, and intellectualization to handle the self-assertive impulses and the anger at frustration). "I don't know" is likely to be the first answer that comes to her lips when she is questioned on practically any topic. This reply is not simply employed to avoid self-incrimination; it is often a fact, for memories are frequently not accessible to such a child, and when they are, they are vague and impressionistic. The most disturbed and immature child (on the histrionic personality pole) has the most primitive defenses, including splitting or dissociation, projection, somatization, passive aggression, and withdrawal into fantasy.

TREATMENT

The optimal treatment is psychoanalytic treatment or expressive psychoanalytic psychotherapy to resolve the conflicts around dependence and sexual inhibitions due to guilt over incestuous wishes. Addressing issues of rivalry and envy affecting friendship and love relationships also are goals in the treatment.

At times, only a trial of treatment will differentiate between the more seriously ill child, with her immature defenses and intense parental stimulation, and the less-disordered child, whose defenses are dominated by repression with greater concealment behind her symptoms. Although it may be that the more neurotic child can be successfully treated alone, family therapy with the parents is a great adjunct for a good outcome in the more severe types.

Techniques of psychoanalytic psychotherapy for children with borderline personality organization are applicable to children with hysterical features.

The techniques are anchored in the integration of a cohesive, stable self, the resolution of primitive defenses, and active work on peer relations. Once these goals are achieved, work on the sexual conflicts and narcissistic defenses can take place as elucidated in the chapter on narcissistic personality disorder.

III.3

Avoidant Personality Disorder

DEFINITION

According to *DSM-IV*, the essential feature of avoidant personality disorder is a pervasive pattern of social inhibition, feelings of inadequacy, and hypersensitivity to negative evaluation that begins by early adulthood and is present in a variety of contexts. Diagnostic criteria include:

avoidance of school or work activities involving significant interpersonal contact because of fears of criticism, disapproval, or rejection;

reluctance or refusal to accept promotions or new relationships for fear of potential criticism or rejection by others;

the conviction that others are critical and disapproving, and the need for nurturance, repeated offers of support, and assurance of uncritical acceptance;

demonstration of restraint, difficulty talking about the self, and withholding of intimate feelings for fear of being exposed, ridiculed, or shamed;

low threshold for detecting such criticism or disappointment;

the view of the self as socially inept, personally unappealing, or inferior to others; and

a reluctance to take on personal risks (either physical or social) or to engage in any new activities.

DSM-IV notes that avoidant PD appears equally in both males and females and has a prevalence in the population between 0.5 and 1.0 percent. Although cautioning the reader to use the diagnosis carefully in children and adolescents for whom shy and avoidant behavior may be developmentally appropriate, the manual indicates that onset "often starts in infancy or childhood with shyness, isolation, and fear of strangers or new situations"(*DSM-IV*, p. 633).

AVOIDANT PERSONALITY DISORDER IN CHILDREN

The substantial literature on avoidance behavior from infancy through adulthood generally views it as an isolated trait rather than as a PD. Several studies have recognized avoidant PDs in adolescents but combined adult subjects in the sample, precluding the drawing of further distinctions between the age groups (Llopis Sala and Gomez Benyto 1994, Rodriguez Torres and Del Porto 1995, Naziroglu et al. 1996). Avoidance behavior has been found to be more prevalent in otherwise physically or psychiatrically compromised children and adolescents than in their so-called normal peers; for example, it appeared at a higher rate among anorexic and bulimic patients than among normal dieters (Keck and Fiebert 1986). C. Last (1989) differentiated anxiety disorders in childhood into separation, avoidant, and overanxious disorders, but she did not view the avoidance behavior as part of an overall personality organization. Instead, she treated the three diagnostic categories, included in *DSM-III*, as differing in the specific focus of the anxiety.

The origins of avoidant PD are also discussed with respect to temperament in developmental research. A. Matheny (1989) described his longitudinal study of 130 twins from 12 to 30 months and reported that his results affirm "temperament characteristics" that characterize some children as upset, shy, or withdrawn when faced with unfamiliar or unexpected circumstances. C. Strauss (1990) also conducted a longitudinal study of childhood anxiety disorders and reported that differential diagnosis can be applied to three subtypes: separation anxiety, overanxious, and avoidant. The study noted both continuity and discontinuity of avoidant behavior in childhood in the histories of adults who present with anxiety disorders. J. Kagan and N. Snidman (1991) observed that the initial dispositions to approach or avoid unfamiliar events appears moderately stable over time, on the basis of a longitudinal study from age 4 months to age 2 years.

The duration of avoidance depends on the degree of initial intensity. D. Hamilton and N. King (1991) administered the Behavioral Avoidance Test to children (ages 2–11) with dog phobias, at baseline and one week after, without treatment. Small gains occurred only in the children with relatively mild fears, suggesting that children with more pervasive fears do not improve spontaneously. Severity may indicate an underlying personality disturbance that does not allow for spontaneous recovery.

A. Ebata and R. Moos (1994) studied 259 adolescents (ages 12–18) and noted correlates of avoidant coping style, including greater susceptibility to distress, more chronic stressors, and more experience of negative life events in the previous year. Avoidant coping style in the previous year also predicted avoidant coping one year later.

Some researchers do not find evidence either of distinct forms of avoidance or of avoidant behavior free from developmental variations. G. Francis and her colleagues (1992) initiated a study of children aged 6 years to 17 years to ascertain whether avoidant PDs and social phobia are indeed discrete entities. G. Francis and F. D'Elia (1994) reviewed the empirical data available and questioned whether children diagnosed with avoidant PD who also exhibit significant social anxiety can be considered to have a distinct avoidant PD. P. Kahlbaugh and J. Haviland (1986) investigated nonverbal behavior and avoidance behaviors in families with children aged 7–16 during a family interaction task. The results indicate increased avoidance in early adolescents in the form of shame and increased avoidance in the older adolescents in the form of contempt. Increased avoidance as a function of age was supported by the overall data.

The contradictory findings in the literature may be a function of the lack of a shared conceptualization of avoidance and whether it is a state or trait; whether it is dependent or independent of development, situational factors, and environmental stressors; whether it is a symptom that may range from normal to pathological; and whether it is related or unrelated to other aspects of personality. In our view, avoidant PD does apply to children and adolescents and can be distinguished from situational and/or developmental avoidant behavior.

The definition in *DSM-IV* readily translates into childhood equivalents. Children with avoidant PD are characterized by avoidance of school or extracurricular activities (such as not trying out for a theater production or competitive sports team because of fears of criticism, disapproval, or rejection). Peer relations and friendships are adversely affected because these children are unwilling to get involved with others unless they are unconditionally accepted. Like their adult counterparts, these children are consumed with anxiety about what their peers think, and they expect to be criticized or rejected. They tend to be emotionally constricted and laconic for fear of saying the wrong thing and sounding foolish or being ridiculed. Transitions to new schools, neighborhoods, or classrooms are particularly inhibiting for them because of their conviction of personal inadequacy, and taking personal risks, such as participating in a play or having a public role in a school function, is overwhelming.

DIFFERENTIAL DIAGNOSIS

Differential diagnosis requires the application of criteria for avoidant PD. Does the child's avoidant behavior appear to be enduring and present during different phases of life, or even during a period of a year? Does it have an inflexible, rigid, and maladaptive quality that leaves the child unable to overcome challenging situations and move on from them?

Avoidant behavior may be seen in a temperamentally shy child who lacks self-confidence about his performance or social acceptability. The shy child is slow to warm up but is able to master the situation given support, time, and increased familiarity. The shy child's lack of experience does not necessarily imply a chronic conviction of inadequacy that has to be protected, as typified by the child with avoidant PD.

Clinically, avoidant behavior needs to be differentiated from schizoid PD, which evidences more social detachment and aloofness along with emotional constriction and preference for solitary experiences, not out of fear of rejection but out of indifference toward, and lack of pleasure in, social interactions. Children and adolescents with paranoid symptomatology will also experience anxiety and avoidance in social situations but in a different context: Other people are the objects of suspiciousness and mistrust, with the potential for malevolence.

The concept of avoidant PD in children would subsume social phobia and aspects of separation anxiety. When discussing differential diagnosis between avoidant PD and social phobia, generalized, *DSM-IV* observes that they overlap extensively and that both can be included in a diagnosis. In referring to that overlap when defining avoidant PD, however, it states that the two "may be alternative conceptualizations of the same or similar conditions" (pp. 663–664).

Significant distinctions do exist in the nature of the social interaction with others. The individual with avoidant PD requires stringent proof that others will be supportive, nurturing, and noncritical in order to tolerate any engagement with others. From the cognitive/perceptual standpoint, whereas someone with social phobia, generalized type, automatically fears social situations where he might embarrass himself, the individual with avoidant PD has a heightened vigilance for any possible criticism or rejection. The search for subtle or even deceptive cues of disapproval and the misinterpretation of another's social cues is distinct from the general belief (or fear) that certain social situations will lead to criticism, rejection, or humiliation.

In their comprehensive review of generalized social phobia and its relation to avoidant PD, D. Beidel and S. Turner (1997) observe that onset of the former before age 11 predicts nonrecovery as an adult. From their literature review, they conclude that individuals with generalized social phobia, in contrast to specific phobias, have more severe symptoms of shyness and a history of greater incidence, a family social style characterized by social isolation, greater neuroticism, and more introversion. The authors also conclude that the findings of earlier onset and greater severity indicate a qualitative difference between generalized social phobia and specific subtypes of phobia.

Beidel and Turner argue that generalized social phobia represents a chronic social inadequacy that is related to avoidant PD, reporting that some 22 percent of adults diagnosed with it also meet the criteria for avoidant PD (Turner et al. 1991). Individuals with generalized social phobia, unlike those with specific social phobia, are deficient in social skills, such as maintaining conversations, listening to others, perceiving social cues, and difficulty actively planning social activities. These deficits suggest "a lag in their social interactions." When avoidant PD is diagnosed comorbidly with social phobia, the clinical picture is more severe with respect to phobic symptomatology, general measures of anxiety, depression, and social functioning.

The distinction between a phobia and a PD is critical because of the implications for treatment. The patient with avoidant PD has a more profound and pervasive investment in confirming her view through "proof" of another's critical cues and actively tries to extract reassurance and support from others. Beidel and Turner note that certain avoidant PD traits meet criteria for obsessive-compulsive PD as well, including perfectionism, overconscientiousness, ethical inflexibility, rigidity, and interpersonal difficulty. The patient with social phobia, generalized, would simply avoid others because of a irrational belief. Beidel and Turner confirm, for example, that patients with avoidant PD do not respond well to intensive treatment using imagery or in vivo exposure; they advise the use of alternative treatments, focusing on social skills training.

Avoidant PD also shares features with generalized anxiety disorder (which includes overanxious disorder of childhood), including the affective experience of worry about competence or quality of performance and apprehensive expectation. The distinction between the two involves the lack of specificity in the generalized anxiety disorder, the absence of a focal anxiety about the other's critical perception of the self, and the attempts to control the anxiety through social avoidance or demands for reassurance. Worries about the safety of family members, financial stability, or potential major repairs of a house or car would not characterize avoidant PD.

Selective mutism (formerly "elective mutism"), a disorder marked by a persistant failure to speak in specific social situations, is also associated with excessive shyness, fear of social embarrassment, social isolation, and withdrawal. This disorder is rare and found in less than one percent of individuals seen in mental health settings, according to *DSM-IV*. The specific nature of the refusal to speak and the absence of the other personality traits noted in avoidant PD allow for a distinction to be made between the two disorders.

The child with avoidant PD differs from the nonpatient peer in his chronic lack of skills or resources for bouncing back; consequently, he fails to achieve eventual mastery of an anxiety-producing situation. All aspects of the personality are affected. Neither the inhibition of emotional expression nor the pattern of avoidance of new activities is consistent with the developmental norm. Unlike their healthier counterparts, children with avoidant PD have chronic feelings of inadequacy that are incompatible with the narcissism of normal development, which embodies optimism about the future and confidence in abilities and social desirability. Continued withdrawal from others, from new opportunities for mastery, and from their own emotional worlds in order to feel safe from the perceived threats of taking risks and getting involved with others commonly generates comorbidity with depression in children with avoidant PD.

COMPARISON WITH ADULT
AVOIDANT PERSONALITY DISORDER

There is little discontinuity between children and adults with avoidant PD except that the status of a school child is not affected as that of a worker may be by the pathological wariness to accept new job situations or transitions. Peer relations, involvement in new activities, emotional restriction, and self-concept are likely to be similar in presentation. The adverse impact on social interactions interferes with the establishment of intimate, long-term relationships in adults, which would not be applicable to children.

DEVELOPMENTAL PSYCHOPATHOLOGY

The development of shyness, avoidant reactions, difficulty with transitions, and apprehension when exposed to new stimuli has been posited to begin at birth in the form of genetic and constitutional factors. J. Kagan and N. Snidman (1991) studied youngsters from 10 months to 10 years of age and noted the continuity of a well-defined syndrome of early clinginess and extreme shyness in certain children in their inhibited behavior around strangers during later development. Kagan and Snidman report that even though the behavior was not insensitive to development, it could be identified as a common process that manifested itself across different developmental periods.

At age 3, children show anxiety about physical harm, loss of parental love, being different, or not being able to cope with events. C. E. Schaefer and H. L. Millman (1994) observe that typical signs of anxiety include agitation, crying, screaming, pacing, obsessive thinking, insomnia, nightmares, poor eating, sweating, "butterflies in the stomach," nausea, breathing difficulties, and tics. They distinguish between the anxious child, typically between the ages of 2 and 6, with weak distinctions between reality and fantasy, and "highly anxious" children of the same age whose behavior is more inflexible and rigid. The "highly anxious" child is less popular, less creative, more suggestible, indecisive, and cautious. The personality is marked by poor self-image, greater dependency on adults, and lower scores on intelligence and achievement tests. Although the authors do not use the term "personality disorder," the features described are consistent with avoidant PD. Children with physical or cognitive deficits appear to be more at risk, given their awareness of being different from and possibly less capable than others.

Environment contributes to the development of further avoidance behavior through the mother/infant interaction, family factors, environmental stressors on the family, and trauma endured in the first few years of life. M. Stone (1993) observes that environmental influences are not only important but also sufficient in generating avoidant PD. Children can be "programmed" to fear and avoid many kinds of persons and situations most people consider harmless. Generational influence may pass down the disorder through an anxious, avoidant parent. Stone also covered other environmental factors, including such traumatic patterns as parental brutalization, incest, and sexual molestation in childhood. Schaefer and Millman (1994) also include parental criticism, perfectionism, neglect, or involving the child as an adult confidante.

Avoidant personality traits are self-reinforcing because of the immediate relief from anxiety that strengthens and perpetuates the condition.

TREATMENT

Treatment of avoidant PD includes both cognitive and behavioral interventions in the form of social skills training, exposure to feared situations, enhancement of problem-solving, ability to develop coping mechanisms other than avoidance, and training in anxiety management in the face of dreaded situations. Beidel and Turner (1997) include the treatment goal of accepting some uncertainty regarding the actions of others when engaging in social interactions. They urge pediatric clinicians to help their younger patients to understand the rationale behind exposure to the feared situation as being a useful way to overcome fears.

Psychoanalytic approaches explore underlying conflicts that lead to compromised behavior, such as unconscious oedipal and pre-oedipal fears of being separated from mother, conflicts with aggression and unconscious destructive or aggressive fantasies and impulses, or risking rivalry with father by being successful in competition. Exploration of the function of the avoidant traits may also reveal underlying grandiose self-images that the individual fears must be kept under wraps so as not to overwhelm others. Similarly, embarrassment and inhibition about sexual or exhibitionistic impulses may underlie the need to be avoidant and vigilant about potentially mortifying exposure.

Pharmacological interventions reduce the child's reactivity, allowing for tolerance of anxiety and the better use of treatment.

CLINICAL EXAMPLE

Tom, a 13-year-old adolescent, came in for an evaluation because of his pervasive avoidance of engagement with others, particularly with his male peers; his inhibited behavior in sporting events; his quiet, unresponsive relationship with his family members; and his persistent preoccupation that his clothing would be criticized by others. Tom explained that he would hold back from shooting baskets because people might think that he was showing off and would make fun of him if he missed when they thought he expected to make it.

Tom presented as emotionally constricted but was able to acknowledge that his avoidant activity and preoccupation with being perceived as not fitting into the group was painful to him. His mother also presented with a history of fearfulness, avoidance, and social loneliness, whereas his father was absorbed with work and physically and emotionally unavailable to Tom. Tom's cluelessness about his internal world of thoughts and feelings left him feeling adrift in his interactions with others, wanting desperately to be accepted and successful but convinced that he would be exposed as not worthwhile. Tom agreed that his life did not have to continue in this manner and was amenable to seeking treatment.

Brief psychological screening using the Rorschach Inkblot Test, the Thematic Apperception Test, and the Achenbach Child Behavior Checklist (CBCL) indicated consistent personality features that contributed to the avoidant PD diagnosis. The CBCL, which measures the parents' perception of the child, revealed mild somatic complaints and tendencies to withdraw and be secretive. The Anxious/Depressed Index was at the borderline pathological level and included such symptoms as feeling worthless, self-conscious, anxious, and inadequate. The Rorschach profile was positive on the Coping Deficit Index, which is associated with chronically inept, ineffective responses to interpersonal situations.

Tom's Rorschach Test response was emblematic of a teenager living on the periphery of the social world, observing but not participating. The signs of Tom's social isolation, his distortion of reality, his immature and fantasy-based representations of self and others, and his inability to engage with others in an emotional manner, whether aggressively or cooperatively, were consistent with the expectable implications of having avoidant PD. Its cognitive underpinnings are exemplified in Tom's severe narrowing of his perceptions into simplistic, black-and-white formulations. He also evidenced the tendency to scan his world hastily and haphazardly and to jump to conclusions that would likely be inaccurate or unexpected by others. His vulnerability to misinterpreting his experiences was significant. Tom could easily misconstrue the world in a way that conformed to his previous expectations and reinforce the need to respond in the same avoidant way.

After the testing feedback was shared with Tom, he decided that he would like to work on his issues by himself. He realized that he needed to take more risks and not to care so much about others' opinions. He agreed to return in a few months if he did not make progress. Not surprisingly, the issue of entering into treatment is an obstacle in itself for children and adolescents like Tom, whose avoidant PD may, ironically, keep them away from the very situation that could potentially help them.

III.4

Obsessive-Compulsive
Personality Disorder

DEFINITION

DSM-IV defines Obsessive-Compulsive Personality Disorder (OCPD) as "a preoccupation with orderliness, perfectionism and mental and interpersonal control, at the expense of flexibility, openness, and efficiency" (p. 285). Although it notes that the pattern begins by early adulthood, *DSM-IV* neither reviews the origins of OCPD nor makes reference to its onset in children. Diagnostic criteria follow:

- preoccupation with details, rules, lists, order, organization, or schedules to the extent that the major point of the activity is lost;
- perfectionism that interferes with task completion;
- excessive devotion to work and productivity, to the exclusion of leisure activities and friendships; and
- overconscientiousness and inflexibility about matters of morality, ethics, or values, independent of culture and religion.

DESCRIPTION

The personality features are often ego-syntonic. OCPD patients are comfortable with their personality characteristics and contemptuous of others' frivolity and impulsivity. They tend to be stilted and morally rigid and easily upset if not in control of their environment. Their emotional expression is compromised by avoidance of anger and discomfort with emotional exchanges. They have difficulty with empathy and with acknowledging others' points of view. The inability to compromise and the insistence that things be done "the right way" alienates them from others. Decision-making and prioritizing become time-consuming and laborious.

OCPD IN CHILDREN

The traits of overcontrol and inhibition of expression of aggression are clinically observed to be compensatory defenses against the underlying sadistic thoughts and fantasies. The underbelly of pleasurably charged raw aggression is readily seen in the play and in the dreams of OCPD children, in dramatic contrast to their constricted behavior in public. The presence of this sadistic material in turn generates further anxiety and amplifies the need both to control others omnipotently and to constrict their own affects internally and interpersonally. (The omnipotent control itself has a sadistic quality, connected to the underlying fears and fantasies.) These behaviors alienate others, adversely impacting friendships and family relationships.

The traits have correlates in normal development, including the deployment of "magical thinking" in the attempt to control others and the hypersensitivity to criticism that children aged 5 to 12 display when questioned. The normal school-aged child is also invested in rules and orderly procedures in games but does not exhibit an oversensivity to "things being just so" and can quickly get over routine disruptions and disappointments. In contrast, the OCPD child can become overwhelmed with rage and/or anxiety when thwarted or frustrated in her attempts to maintain control over both the environment and her own internal states as well.

DIFFERENTIAL DIAGNOSIS

According to several reports, patients diagnosed with OCPD do not necessarily meet the criteria of Obsessive-Compulsive Disorder, which involves the presence of obsessions and compulsions, such as unwanted, senseless, repetitive rituals. Although OCPD is relatively common among patients with OCD, it is considered an independent diagnostic category. G. Diaferia and her research group (1997) analyzed the relationship between OCPD and OCD: They concluded that the two entities may share phenomenological characteristics but do not belong to the same genetic spectrum. They proposed that some OCPD traits may be related to behavioral and lifestyle changes induced by the clinical symptoms of OCD rather than to preexisting personality features. They found no difference in age of onset between OCD patients with OCPD versus those without, and they noted that OCPD was diagnosed in patients as young as 10 years of age.

Patients respond differently to pharmacological interventions when both OCD and OCPD are diagnosed; consequently, it is critical that the latter be identified even in the presence of the former. P. Cavedini and colleagues (1997) reported that the overlap of OCPD with OCD (noted in 31 percent of their OCD sample) predicted poorer response to pharmacological treatment. M. Flament and colleagues (1990) followed 25 inpatients aged 6 to 18 who were diagnosed with OCD: Within two to seven years, 15 children were additionally diagnosed with a PD, five of those (20 percent) with OCPD.

The concept of OCPD in children, even though not acknowledged by *DSM-IV*, is alive in the literature as a focus of researchers and clinicians. Z. Parker and E. Stewart (1994) observed that certain of the traits in children adversely affect school performance. They noted that the educational system "lauds" such OCPD characteristics as neatness, correctness, competition, self-criticism, and the need to retain control—but these characteristics, when taken to excess, become signals of pathology. OCPD children can engage in unnecessary erasing, redoing, and refusal to accept mistakes; some will tear up their homework in anger and frustration.

Parker and Stewart (1994) investigated the impact of OCPD traits in children in an outpatient program for youths aged 12 through 20. Although generally the presenting symptoms interfering with school performance include worrying, excessive expectations, dissatisfaction with results, competitiveness, procrastination, need for control, and self-criticism, several of Parker and Stewart's cases involved presenting symptoms—depression, tantrums, distress about attending school, and poor achievement—that proved to be related to obsessional habits and preoccupations.

C. E. Schaefer and H. L. Millman (1994) view compulsive, perfectionistic behavior as having a normal developmental course. Children often spend inordinate amounts of time grooming, showering, and preparing their clothing. Children between the ages of 2 and 7 enjoy playing rule-bound games, reciting sayings, and performing rituals. Those between the ages of 8 and 10 commonly have compulsions. The children who develop compulsive personalities are those whose fussiness, orderliness, punctuality, intolerance of mess and dirtiness, and overattention to details take excessive time and interfere with ordinary activities. The authors conclude that adults need to determine whether a child is adaptively balancing his striving for excellence with flexibility and tolerance for realistic failures and difficulties.

DEVELOPMENTAL PSYCHOPATHOLOGY

The traditional struggle over whether OCPD, like other personality disorders, stems from genetic or environmental factors is evident in the literature. G. Andrews and his colleagues (1990) concluded that a significant measure of heritability occurred for OCPD—nearly 50 percent. M. Stone (1993) has observed that even though genetic factors set the personality structure, OCPD is "licked into shape by rearing patterns that overemphasize conformity, neatness, automatic obedience to authority and punitiveness" (p. 348). Environments in which caretakers model fearfulness or engage in sustained conflict and criticism can also produce OCPD reactivity. Moreover, OCPD children may be constitutionally highly reactive to sudden changes in their environment and may react with fixed patterns of behavior.

Even the Harvard Mental Health Letter published in February 1996 notes that PDs such as OCPD arise from a complicated process of inherited dispositions, upbringing, and unique experiences. The temperament of a child is observable in infancy in her mood, activity level, persistence, and tendency to seek or avoid risk. OCPD, according to behavioral theories, is likely to be a product of conditioning and reinforcement or learned behavior. Adults with OCPD (as well as an avoidant or dependent personality) may evidence a low threshold for fear and heightened arousal since childhood. Their symptoms are behaviorally determined so as to avoid and protect the self from intolerable levels of affect or unpleasant stimulation. Characteristics of parents that may contribute to OCPD have not been comprehensively studied. The Harvard Mental Health Letter reports that patients in the anxious cluster of PDs tend to believe that their parents were both overprotective and insufficiently affectionate. Indeed, the likely presence of obsessive traits in the parents of OCPD children is a common assumption.

D. Clark and D. Bolton (1985) noted the lack of rigorous definitions of the concepts and of objective assessment procedures in several clinical reports that found parents in OCPD cases to be strict and overinvolved and to have high expectations for their children. Their own study compared parents of adolescents with obsessive-compulsive traits to parents of adolescents with nonobsessive anxiety disorders, and even though their results partially supported the finding that the former were more likely to have obsessive-compulsive traits than normal, nonpatient adults, the level of such traits in them was not significantly different from the level in the parents of the anxious adolescents. The authors concluded that obsessive-compulsive behavior in parents may contribute to anxiety or neuroticism in their children but does not necessarily contribute specifically to OCPD behavior. Interestingly, however, even in the absence of actual differences between the two groups of parents, the OCPD adolescents *perceived* that theirs sustained higher demands than the parents of the anxious adolescents.

In summary, OCPD does appear to present in consistent ways from childhood to adulthood as though the anxiety about loss of control, perfectionism, preoccupation with order, details, and parsimony remains fixed in the personality, indifferent to time and development.

TREATMENT

Psychodynamic treatment of OCPD seeks to transform maladaptive automatic, ego-syntonic behavior and thought processes compatible with the patient's sense of self into ego-dystonic or incompatible behavior and thought processes that the patient can readily identify, recognize as maladaptive, and then resolve. Psychodynamic approaches focus on the conflict underlying and giving rise to the OCPD trait, toward helping the patient deal with the unacceptable wish and fear in direct, adaptive ways. For example, a child who is troubled by angry, murderous wishes toward a parent may engage in a campaign of unrealistically high moral standards and self-reproaches to ward off his guilt and anxiety.

Analysis of the defense mechanisms used in coping with the anxiety, such as reaction formation, isolation of affects, rationalization, and displacement, should be clarified and interpreted so that the patient is aware of both their existence and their maladaptive consequences. Thus, a child who does not want to go to a birthday party because "it would be boring" would be rationalizing the anxiety triggered by contemplating being in that social situation—and, in addition, denying that anxiety by claiming boredom. In another case, which will be expanded later, a child who maintains an emotionally intense fantasy life by conducting an imaginary newspaper while presenting with a flat and constricted sober affect illustrates the use of displacement from the interpersonal realm to an imaginary realm that he controls. Alternate solutions can be found to liberate the patient from such constricted defensive operations when the fantasy is brought to the surface.

Cognitive/behavioral approaches target the pathological thinking and behavior directly, without delving into the meaning of the behavior. Such models treat OCD/OCPD symptoms through exposure and response prevention, the two principal techniques of reducing pathological behavior. Exposure places the patient in the anxiety-producing situation with increasing frequency and duration until the anxiety or fear subsides; response prevention substitutes a competing or an incompatible behavior or thought for the pathological response. A child whose perfectionism usually leads her to tear up an imperfectly completed assignment, for instance, is taught how to "talk back" to the internal "bully" compelling her to act destructively.

J. March and K. Mulle (1998) have published a systematic manual using cognitive/behavioral techniques to address OCD in children and adolescents. Children are actively enlisted to "do battle" with their symptoms and even to give their symptoms a derogatory name to designate their enemy status. The family serves as cheerleader and does not collude with the "enemy's" attempts to maintain the irrational behavior. Victories are charted and celebrated as the OCD symptoms diminish. March and Mulle's work can be readily applied to OCPD traits that are linked to anxiety or fear, such as perfectionism, hoarding, rumination, indecisiveness, and moral rigidity.

Other traits, particularly emotional constriction, are less accessible to cognitive/behavioral interventions and require intensive, long-term work within the context of a therapeutic relationship or group. The child or adolescent's emotional constriction and avoidance of emotionally charged issues can trigger boredom, fatigue, and irritation in the therapist (Stone 1993) and can require considerable time to resolve. To pave the way for the use of cognitive techniques in preadolescents who have difficulty expressing their thoughts, increasing self-reflective capacity becomes a goal: The therapist seeks to help these patients become aware of what they are thinking when engaging in a particular action.

Treatment of OCPD should integrate individual work with the child, work with the family, and often the school environment. At the school level, Z. Parker and E. Stewart (1994) recommend encouraging the teacher to involve the child in group projects more than in individual work, to emphasize managing one assignment at a time rather than multiple tasks, and to adopt strategies that reduce competitiveness. In addition, school staff can model acceptance of mistakes and prioritize social interaction more than individual contribution. Intellectual assessment is critical to determine the child's actual abilities and identify any learning disabilities that may be contributing to the child's unrealistic expectations and frustrations.

There is no indication for medication for OCPD in the absence of comorbidity. In the cases where OCPD is comorbid with OCD, selected seratonin reuptake inhibitors (SSRIs) are indicated (Cavedini et al. 1997, Flament et al. 1990).

CLINICAL EXAMPLE

Charlie, a 12-year-old boy from a Catholic family, presented with widespread anxiety symptoms. He was preoccupied with the idea of going to hell, guilt-ridden over having stepped on an ant at age 4, and he worried that his having played with matches four months before a school fire occurred indicated a possible culpability. Charlie had difficulty falling asleep because of his ruminations on his own "sinfulness." His parents described him as perfectionistic and "obsessive-compulsive" in his daily habits. Always concerned about his homework, Charlie would cry if he got an A-; he felt compelled to say prayers at specific moments of the day and to count steps as he walked through the kitchen. Although he had some friendships, Charlie was shy: He seemed to take refuge in solitary activities like reading and writing and would remark to his mother that "nothing seems funny to me."

The formal psychological evaluation results were consistent with both OCD and OCPD. Charlie's affect was sober and restrained, and his test behavior was meticulous; performance was generally poorer on timed tests. The Rorschach Test results indicated that he had chronic difficulties managing the everyday demands in his life and was easily unraveled. He tended to misinterpret or distort situations and to develop highly idiosyncratic and overpersonalized conclusions about himself and others. His significant neglect of details and nuances left him susceptible to jumping to conclusions and to interpreting situations in black-or-white ways—to reducing anything complex or ambiguous into its most simplistic version. Charlie's overly moralistic and perfectionistic stance left him devoid of pleasure, and his emotional functioning was in keeping with his presentation: He failed to give any color responses to the chromatic inkblots in the Rorschach cards, and this extremely unusual omission correlates with a massive restriction of affect and an inability to identify or express affect adaptively.

Also consistent with OCPD was the presence of a tendency to ruminate about negative aspects of the self. Charlie also appeared to be socially isolated or engaged at a superficial level with others. His own self-image was quite poor. His common way of handling anxiety, the protocol suggested, was to avoid taking responsibility for or to avoid initiating action until someone else could take care of the problem. Of particular concern was his escaping into fantasy to an excessive degree to avoid the discomfort of pressures or problems. During the initial course of treatment, Charlie's capacity to delve into private fantasy contrasted markedly to his constricted ability to convey everyday interactions and feelings about others.

Charlie's sessions revealed a tumultuous fantasy life that was tightly controlled in the form of a fictional newspaper. The newspaper would report events about rock stars being assaulted by thugs and the school walls being broken down by out-of-control criminal elements. Juxtaposed with this newspaper was a repetitive and carefully detailed drawing of the weekly movie marquee that listed 10 movies. Charlie was drawn to using bright colors and vivid contrasts, but only in a predictable and stylized way. As he drew, he would talk about his worries as to whether he would go to heaven; the therapy would attempt to integrate the world of fantasy with his anxiety about possible repercussions.

The work proceeded very slowly, and Charlie's family was referred for psychiatric consultation to evaluate pharmacological interventions. He was diagnosed as being depressed along with having OCD, and he was given Prozac. Charlie did not return to therapy.

After seven years, he was contacted to see if he would come for a follow-up interview and a Rorschach evaluation. Charlie, now 19 years old, agreed, and he brought three stories he had written during college. These stories, fictional accounts from the perspective of a doctor and a physically abused nurse, were intensely emotional and passionate. The passion, however, was completely contained in the internal thoughts of the characters and not in their interaction, which was marked by constraint and wariness about revealing true feelings. Charlie's manner was equally subdued and sober, in contrast to the colorful material, as he described his current life.

He still lived at home with his parents and attended college. He "hung out" at a study hall where he would socialize with some other students who did not live on campus, and he still preferred, as he had seven years earlier, to engage in solitary pursuits, such as writing, in his leisure time. He was no longer anxious about heaven and hell, but he did feel he was more conscientious than others about getting homework done and thinking about assignments during the weekends. He denied any OCD behavior. When asked how he was perceived by others, he replied that friends described him as always being serious. He did not have any interest in establishing a romantic relationship and felt that he did not seem to have the sexual desires of his peers. Charlie felt that his life was satisfactory and did not wish to change any aspect of it; he was curious, however, about what another Rorschach Test would indicate and how the results would compare to those of the earlier one.

The second Rorschach Test confirmed the continuation of several of the first Rorschach's findings, including the chronic inability to handle such everyday demands as managing interpersonal conflicts; balancing time for self with time for others, schoolwork, and family; and effectively dealing with normal emotional reactions (frustration, anger, resentment). The results also indicated a tendency to neglect subtle cues and nuances, limiting him to hasty, inaccurate conclusions about the world, a further avoidance of emotionally laden situations, and a worsened self-image. He still used (or abused) fantasy excessively to avoid dealing with painful or difficult situations and continued to ruminate negatively about himself. The nature of these fantasies, as suggested by his stories and the Rorschach content, often involved aggression toward others or preoccupation with a damaged sense of self. The story characters were all emotionally damaged as well as abused. Charlie appeared to live vicariously through the roles of the victimizer and the victim, both of whom he identified with in his aggressive, emotionally charged dramas.

The differences between the two Rorschachs were also informative, given that Charlie had gone through adolescence without the benefit of any treatment. He still related to others in a superficial way or remained on the periphery of social interactions, but he was less socially isolated. His tolerance for emotional experience shifted from a complete absence to a limited capacity to acknowledge and to express feelings. Charlie's ability to view his world accurately was significantly improved, but he was also feeling more depressed. Cognitive constriction (or possibly defensiveness) was apparent in his giving only 14 responses, compared with 23 when he was 12; 23 is average. The constriction could be viewed as the aftermath of several OCPD defensive operations: Charlie had to censor and suppress the inkblots' evocative aspects by controlling his responses quantitatively and qualitatively. His choosing not to see what was possible to see indicates the use of denial; his avoidance of the affectively charged chromatic cards evidences isolation, whereby thoughts are stripped of disturbing or distressing emotions.

Charlie's case suggests that development by itself did not significantly resolve the earlier personality traits underlying the OCPD. The nature of his PD underwent transformation, however, and would not likely be called OCPD in its current presentation. Charlie's adaptation appears more schizoid in nature and lacks the distinguishing OCPD traits—the perfectionism, the preoccupation with moral virtue, the relentless ruminations about guilt, and the compulsion to order and contain his inner life—that characterized him earlier. Rather, consistent with a schizoid PD, he has shifted to a solitary life. His superficial contacts with others are a way of managing the demands of his own emotional life and of social interactions in general. The fictional newspaper underwent a transformation into fictional stories about pained and angry adults, his current refuge for coping with unacceptable or too intense emotional exchanges.

Without treatment, Charlie developed another PD as a young adult that continued to interfere severely with his adjustment. The case of Charlie illustrates that recognition of the enduring traits underlying OCPD as they first appear in childhood, and development of a long-term treatment strategy that educates the child and the family about the symptoms not touched by medication alone, need to be incorporated in clinical theory and practice.

PART IV
THE BORDERLINE
PERSONALITY ORGANIZATION

IV.1

Introduction

Borderline personality organization (O. Kernberg 1975, 1996) subsumes the Cluster B personality disorders—borderline, narcissistic, histrionic, and antisocial—that are distinguished by:

Identity disturbance or identity diffusion. A chronic unstable image of the self in terms of cohesiveness; intentionality; constancy across time and situations; autonomy; gender; and ethical, cultural, and ideological values;

Primitive defense mechanisms based on splitting. Projective identification, denial, primitive idealization, devaluation, omnipotent control—all of which underlie impairments in impulse control; affect regulation; and tolerance for frustration, anxiety, and depression so serious that they interfere with adaptation to external and internal reality; and

Preservation of the capacity to maintain contact with reality in spite of regression and micropsychotic episodes.

Borderline personality disorder (BPD), whose hallmark is a chaotic and reckless life, is characterized by unstable, intense relations, impulsivity, anger, identity disturbance, and suicidal behaviors. Described as consistently inconsistent, BPD patients rely on the entire constellation of defense mechanisms centered on splitting.

In narcissistic personality disorder (NPD), the borderline organization appears to be more stable as a result of the masking effects of the defining grandiose self. The grandiose self is the result of blending realistic perceptions of the self with the ego ideal, the ideal self, and the ideal objects. It causes pathology in the regulation of self-esteem because the grandiose self demands constant feedback in the form of unconditional admiration from others to maintain the belief that it is the most perfect and powerful. The devalued self is split off, and its vulnerability to the slightest frustration is obscured—yet the patient is subject to rage storms because of the disequilibrium of the grandiose self vis-à-vis reality. Splitting and related mechanisms are present, but devaluation is the key defense mechanism.

Histrionic personality disorder (HPD) is essentially the extreme pole of the hysterical spectrum; as such, it is elucidated in conjunction with the hysterical personality (neurotic personality organization). Antisocial personality disorder (ASPD) combines narcissistic PD with a conduct disorder.

IV.2

Borderline Personality Disorder

DEFINITION

Borderline Personality Disorder as defined by *DSM-IV* is a pervasive pattern of instability in interpersonal relationships, self-image, and affects, together with a marked impulsivity beginning by early adulthood and present in a variety of contexts, as indicated by five (or more) of the following:

frantic efforts to avoid real or imagined abandonment;

a pattern of unstable and intense interpersonal relationships characterized by alternating between extremes of idealization and devaluation;

identity disturbance—markedly and persistently unstable self-image or sense of self;

impulsivity in at least two areas that are potentially self-damaging (e.g., spending, sex, substance abuse, reckless driving, binge eating);

recurrent suicidal behavior, gestures, or threats, or self-mutilating behavior;

affective instability due to a marked reactivity of mood (e.g., intense episodic dysphoria, irritability, or anxiety usually lasting a few hours and only rarely more than a few days);

chronic feeling of emptiness;

inappropriate, intense anger or difficulty controlling anger (e.g., frequent displays of temper, constant anger, recurrent physical fights); and

transient, stress-related paranoid ideation or severe dissociative symptoms.

DESCRIPTION

In children, borderline PD is characterized by the persistence of multiple neurotic and behavioral symptoms—including obsessions, phobias, compulsions, and hysterical traits—that should have been outgrown.

The challenge of differential diagnosis is to distinguish normal transitory developmental symptoms and traits from the multiple severe symptomatology of the borderline patient. During adolescence specifically, depression, anxiety, identity crisis (with its rapid shifts of identification with a certain social group or ideology), neurotic conflicts with authority, even activations of primitive defensive operations like occasionally antisocial behavior and infantile narcissistic object relations have neither the severity and chronicity in the normal teenager that they do in the borderline one. The same is true of younger children.

The case of Jane, a 9-year-old outpatient with signs of ADHD, highlights some of the characteristics just outlined. Jane, who lived with her parents and two older siblings (ages 11 and 12), came to the outpatient department because of attentional problems, awkwardness, and some "social problems." Her teachers were concerned about her poor academic progress; her isolation from her peers, who did not include her in games; and her tendency to give either incorrect or seemingly unrelated answers to questions in class. Jane had become increasingly reluctant to go to school, saying that the other children made fun of her and called her names.

At home, Jane was afraid to be alone. She had nightmares and was terrified of the dark, fearing monsters would enter her room. For two months preceding the evaluation, she had slept in the same bed with her father; earlier, she had slept in her mother's room. She was preoccupied with fears that her parents or her pet guinea pig would die.

Sometimes Jane talked with people "who were not there," although her mother indicated that these were not clearly distinct characters. Frequently, she mumbled or made up words. She had temper tantrums and was very jealous of her sisters, fighting a great deal with them both verbally and physically. She liked to wear boys' clothing, particularly Cub Scouts uniforms, and wanted to put on exactly the same things after school every day.

Born by cesarean section, Jane was described as a difficult baby who cried, "never slept," and spit up frequently. Yet she liked to be held. She sat at 6 months, walked at 11 months, and spoke single words at 8 or 9 months and sentences at 1 year. She was easily toilet trained by age 2. Starting nursery school presented difficulties because Jane was afraid of her teacher. Although she adjusted, she was frequently absent for illness. In the third grade she began to say she did not want to go to school.

Jane's mother was described as having the same fears as her daughter. She was, for instance, fascinated by monster movies and watched them frequently. When her husband had to work at night, she would take the children and sleep at the maternal grandmother's house because she did not like to stay alone overnight, indicating a confusion of generational boundaries. The marriage was described as "working well," although father and mother slept in different quarters and the patient with one or the other.

Clinically, Jane seemed of normal intelligence even though she was functioning 6 months below grade level. With the interviewer, she talked continually and showed a full range of affect, but her speech was tangential or digressive. Although she knew the names of the days of the week, she did not know how many there were. In listing the months of the year, she skipped one and also once went out of sequence. She was aware that she tended to mix up days, months, and years but blamed her classmates for her shortcomings. Nevertheless, there were no loose associations, nor was there evidence of delusions or hallucinations.

Jane described herself as small and ugly and complained that other children picked on her. Her use of primitive defense mechanisms was illustrated in her comment that she was angry with a classmate and wanted to bite him. "But," she added, "I don't want bite marks." When asked how she would get bite marks, she explained that biting people leaves marks. She denied that she thought her classmate would bite her in return. Although she was patient with the interviewer's questions, she was unable to clarify how she instead of her classmate would end up with bite marks.

At another point Jane explained that for awhile she had been afraid that most of her dreams would come true but had learned this was not so. Once she dreamed that a monster would attack her house, and she spent the following day waiting in terror. When no monster appeared, she concluded that monster dreams did not come true; she also remembered her mother's telling her that these dreams were not real.

In the family diagnostic interview, it was apparent that the family behaved in an enmeshed way, with little distinction of generational boundaries. Jane seemed to be used as the joker in the family to divert the focus of any emotionally charged topic. She also tended to cling to her mother and allowed herself to be treated as the baby in the family.

Psychological test reports indicated a full IQ of 96 on the WISC-R (Verbal IQ 90, Performance IQ 105). Jane's language problems were particularly evident in word-finding difficulties. She also showed problems with auditory memory, having trouble remembering the questions. (The impairment in auditory memory was also seen in the Auditory Sequential Memory Test of the Illinois Test of Psycholinguistic Abilities, on which she scored at the 8.8 age level.)

The overall diagnostic impression from neurological and psychological testing was of temporal parietal lobe left hemisphere dysfunction, characterized by short-term auditory memory, word-finding difficulties, letter and number sequence reversals, and trouble with borrowing and carrying in arithmetic. There was the suggestion of a mild right-sided involvement of the left-hand side. In addition, in some of her verbalizations, Jane seemed to confuse active and passive. She also showed trouble following directions, apparently because of attention difficulties and problems in expressing herself verbally.

On projective testing, Jane relied on projection as a defense, indicating, for example, that her mother was a "murderous person." Love and acceptance could never be obtained from mother, who preferred boys and kids who never fought. Jane's protocol was filled with a sense of bleakness, inner impoverishment, and helplessness. Fantasies of running away from the bad mother were intense, as were death fantasies.

Jane had a core female gender identity but showed considerable gender identity confusion. Her wish to be a boy was related to her belief that her mother valued boys and thought girls were useless. In addition, her boyishness seemed to be a defense against very intense and exciting sexual feelings for her father, who was seen as a good person but unavailable to her.

A reason for Jane's distancing herself from people could be discerned in intense aggressive impulses that threatened to overwhelm her and destroy the object. On the Rorschach Test, for instance, she saw two women who were on the verge of ripping apart a crab but were kept from doing so by a butterfly. The butterfly seemed to symbolize the weakness of her ego to defend against the aggressive impulses. Other responses on the projective tests were not well related to the percepts on the cards. Her protocol suggested a chronic borderline structure with a long-standing withdrawal into an idiosyncratic world. There were many peculiar verbalizations, a tendency toward contamination, and a few instances of loss of reality testing when she felt overwhelmed by aggression.

Following *DSM -IV* criteria, Jane was given a diagnosis of separation anxiety disorder, developmental disorder, and mixed personality disorder with borderline personality organization. The underlying borderline personality organization can be seen in a number of areas. Jane clearly showed the poor peer relations, uneven early development, and deficits in academic performance characteristic of borderline children. Difficult sibling relationships were also present. Her dyadic relationship with her parents could be seen in her sleeping habits. Particularly telling was the uncertain identity and unstable self-concept evident in Jane's inability to be alone, her dressing in boys' clothing, and her confusion about whether to play the baby or the clown in the family. She also showed a tendency toward paranoid ideation, as well as the persistence of fears and symptoms beyond the age-appropriate stage. Yet her capacity to test reality was preserved. Finally, it is important to note the role of organicity in complicating Jane's problems. Her problems in word-finding, spatial sequencing, and short-term auditory memory contributed to frustrating experiences with her mother, increasing aggression and interfering with her process of separation/individuation.

The case of Jane underlines the need to assess borderline PD descriptively, developmentally, and structurally. Most characteristic are signs of identity disorder and shifting ego states. Organicity and depression are also frequently present, complicating the picture. Only a thorough assessment will indicate which treatments—long-term psychological intervention, medication for such target symptoms as depression, and educational learning approaches—are called for.

COMPARATIVE PERSPECTIVES

We can assume that borderline adults represent chronologically older borderline adolescents. The adult borderline does not differ substantially from the adolescent except in the accrual of secondary complications in the course of living (marriage, children, career vicissitudes), which do not essentially modify the borderline personality organization. Because of the persistence of primitive defense mechanisms (such as splitting and its related defenses) with ongoing ego-weakening effects, the patient has an inability to integrate experience because of incomplete, distorted relations with external objects. The chronic instability of unintegrated superego components deprives the patient of guidelines for the self- and other-evaluation and hence of a stable sense of identity. Therefore, basically unaffected by positive life circumstances, she cannot learn from experience: Time has stopped for the patient. (Consider the example of the 45-year-old woman who acknowledged quite candidly that she just did not feel her age; she felt she was either a little girl or at the most a budding adolescent. Three marriages, four children, a college education, and wide travels throughout the world had not left much of an imprint on her.)

Recently, various studies have focused on the descriptive symptomatology of the borderline personality organization in children (Bemporad et al. 1982, Aarkrog 1981, P. Kernberg 1983, Kestenbaum 1983, Leichtman and Nathan 1983, Pine 1983, Rinsley 1980b, Vela et al. 1983).* Yet a descriptive picture alone does not suffice for understanding the childhood syndrome (Gualtieri et al. 1983).

F. C. Verhulst (1984) tested a set of 28 variables elicited from the literature to determine which ones distinguish borderline children from neurotic and psychotic children. Several proved to be highly sensitive and specific in the borderline/neurotic differentiation: Borderline children were characterized by annihilation anxiety, primary process thinking, shifting levels of ego functioning, identity disturbance, primitive defense mechanisms, micropsychotic states, ineffective superego functioning, oddities of motor functioning, marked fantasy activity, and discrepancy between interest or talent and actual functioning. Withdrawal and its opposite—demanding, clinging, and unpredictable connections—reflected the typical fluctuation of the borderline child's relationships to others. Identity disturbance was considered the single best discriminating item between borderline children, in whom it is present, and neurotic children, in whom it is absent. In contrast, feelings of loneliness, separation anxiety, and hyperactivity did not distinguish borderline children from the neurotic group.

The gap between the borderline and the psychotic groups of children was narrower. Items that most frequently differentiated borderline from psychotic children were demanding, clinging, and unpredictable relationships; primitive defense mechanisms; shifting levels of ego functioning; micropsychotic states; and feelings of loneliness, whereas psychotic children presented more frequently and typically with withdrawn and aloof behavior in their contact with others, need-fulfilling relationships, language and speech

---

*Earlier writings have also contributed to the portrait of the borderline child (see Ekstein and Wallerstein 1954, Frijling-Schreuder 1969, Geleerd 1958, Mahler and Kaplan 1977, Rosenfeld and Sprince 1963, Weil 1953).

peculiarities, special interest or talent in one area, and resistance to change in the environment.

In their discussion, Verhulst and colleagues concluded that demanding, clinging, and unpredictable relations; primitive defense mechanisms; shifting levels of ego functioning; micropsychotic states; and suspicious, paranoid, and marked fantasy activity were mostly sensitive and specific characteristics of borderline children. Even though borderline children can be distinguished from neurotic children, no single item is pathognomonic of them. Characteristically, borderline children show a variety of symptoms covering every area of psychological functioning, including motor functioning (i.e., mild gross motor coordination).

Psychotic children seem to have a more predictable overall functioning, despite their impairment in social and cognitive functioning, which is quite in contrast with the marked fluctuation presented by borderline children and considered almost pathognomonic by J. Bemporad and colleagues (1982). Their study observed that borderline children present with symptoms taken initially for mild or moderate disturbances; only after prolonged diagnostic evaluations or during the course of psychotherapy does the severe pathology become evident. In 42 percent of borderline cases, the psychiatrist needed more time for his or her diagnosis, which was true in only 16 percent of neurotic cases and 26 percent of the psychotic cases.

We not only need to take into account symptoms presented across various diagnostic categories within Axis I of *DSM-IV*, now including specific developmental disorders, but also to address structural and developmental elements. That leads us to consider characteristics that correspond closely to those in Axis II, which encompasses personality traits and personality disorders. Here it is important to note that the child's response to psychological treatment and specific medications will be codetermined by the descriptive syndrome and the underlying personality and developmental learning disorder (Axis II). The prognosis will be more guarded if borderline personality organization is diagnosed as the underlying PD.

In terms of the Axis I diagnosis or descriptive syndrome, we would suspect borderline personality organization in children with Attention Deficit Disorder with hyperactivity; conduct disorder, undersocialized, aggressive; conduct disorder, undersocialized, nonaggressive; and conduct disorder, socialized, aggressive. Yet borderline personality organization may also appear in separation anxiety disorders, overanxious disorders, schizoid disorder of childhood, elective mutism, identity problems, dissociative disorders, and eating disorders, such as anorexia nervosa and bulimia. In addition, specific developmental disorders—reading, arithmetic, or developmental language disorders with or without Attention Deficit Disorder—have all been found in a significant percentage of borderline adolescents and young adults (Andrulonis et al. 1980).

Most clinicians assume that the term "borderline" is not applicable to children because it is generally believed that PDs do not exist in children between 6 and 12 years of age, who are considered to be neurotic, psychotic, or suffering from a behavioral disorder or organic disorder of some sort. *DSM-IV*, however, assumes that if children meet the criteria for a PD of adulthood, they can be so diagnosed. Already, T. A. Petti and W. Law (1981) and J. H. Liebowitz (1981) have demonstrated the applicability of the *DSM-III* diagnosis of adult borderline PD to children in inpatient and outpatient settings, respectively; *DSM-IV* retains those same criteria, per the definition that opens this chapter.

With respect to children, only one reference—Rosenfeld and Sprince 1963—includes identity disturbance, but it is our opinion that a disturbed sense of identity is a crucial diagnostic criterion for borderline personality organization. F. C. Verhulst (1984) substantiates our conviction that it is one of the two most reliable criteria for diagnosing children as borderline, the other being sudden shifts in level of ego functioning. Identity disorder may well be excluded as a criterion in children on the assumption that "identity" is achieved only in adolescence. Initially speaking, this assumption may be so. Yet children between the ages of 6 and 12 have an age-appropriate identity: They *do* have a sense of me-ness. They know who they are and which gender they are. They have a sense of cultural, religious, and ethnic values and a sense of community and group relatedness, as well as a clear idea of their own continuity through various situations and in time. Their awareness of themselves encompasses both objective attributes and subjective experience. Simply put, they know what they can do, what they like, and what they are like.

There is a suggestion of an intrinsic relationship between borderline and affective illness that has been pursued by Schubert and colleagues (1985) in their comparative study of information processing among borderline, major and minor depressive, manic, and schizoaffective patients and normal controls. Borderline patients showed no difference from normal controls in their visual information processing; they were, however, distinct from the patients in the psychotic group in that respect. Interestingly, schizophrenic and schizotypal patients showed impaired visual information processing similar to that of psychotic patients, firmly supporting the separation of schizotypal from borderline PDs.

DEVELOPMENTAL PSYCHOPATHOLOGY

DEVELOPMENTAL ELEMENTS

In assessing borderline PD in children, it is crucial to consider age-appropriate developmental achievements. We find that preschool borderline children have not accomplished certain tasks expected at this age. They cannot tolerate separation from mother, they lack established standards for bad and good, they show an inability to express a wide variety of modulated feelings, and they are uncertain about sexual distinctions. School-aged borderline children are also behind in their developmental achievements. They do not maintain a sense of gender role identity through play or fantasy. Impulse control remains poor, with unpredictable states. These children do not show enjoyment of peer interactions and increased independence from parents, nor do they have a sense of belonging to an extended community. Finally, they have not yet resolved the oedipal complex through sublimatory channels and repression and the achievement of self- and object-constancy.

Turning to developmental milestones expected for preadolescents and adolescents (Senn and Solnit 1968), we see that borderline patients have not acquired a sense of identity or developed age-appropriate abstract thinking. There is little indication of a struggle for emancipation and autonomy from the family, and perceptions of the family tend to be unrealistic. Sex-role identity, with capacity for intimacy and heterosexual adjustment, is not established, and masturbatory fantasies are primarily connected with pregenital themes, such as anal sadistic and oral themes.

A developmental perspective bears on any evaluation of descriptive symptomatology. Various authors point to a characteristic multiple symptomatology, with obsessions, phobias, compulsions, and hysterical traits. (Schizoid personality traits and paranoid personality traits have also been noted in borderline children, but they are relatively less fixed.) It is not, however, the neurotic and behavioral symptoms per se that typify borderline children. What is more characteristic is the reemergence of symptoms that should have been outgrown. Preschool fears and phobias or compulsive behaviors typically found in 2- to 3-year-olds persist, with increasing intensity, beyond these developmental stages. The shifting levels of functioning further confuse the picture, necessitating careful assessment of overall behavior.

The classic prepsychotic personalities—hypomanic, schizoid, and paranoid—are cited in the descriptive symptomatology of borderline conditions. Schizoid personality in children has been described (Pine 1983), but paranoid and hypomanic personalities as understood in adult psychopathology are rare and less fixed in children.

From the developmental perspective, the challenge of differential diagnosis is to distinguish normal transitory developmental symptoms and traits from the multiple severe symptomatology of the borderline patient. In children, BPD is characterized by the persistence of multiple neurotic and behavioral symptoms—including obsessions, phobias, compulsions, and hysterical traits—that should have been outgrown. In adolescents, R. Knight (1953a), O. Kernberg (1975), and R. Grinker and colleagues (1968) have described multiple symptomatology with an assortment of neurotic and character neurotic symptoms (not specific in themselves).

STRUCTURAL ELEMENTS

Recognizing identity disorder and shifting levels of ego organization as fundamental to borderline PD in children and adolescents reflects the application of O. Kernberg's (1978) concept of adult borderline personality organization to our population. Such a structural perspective enables us to understand better the varied symptomatology these children present, both cross-sectionally and in longitudinal studies (Aarkrog 1981, Kestenbaum 1983). The disturbed sense of identity contributes to borderline children's lack of sense of me-ness, their undefined gender identity, and their incapacity to be alone. Their shifting levels of ego function, with abrupt regressions, account for their lack of judgment and their impulsivity, as well as their disturbed relationship to reality. (They can, however, test reality, as per the aforementioned case of Jane: She had seen the movie *Jaws* at the age of 7 when she entered therapy and was afraid to use the toilet because she was afraid "Jaws" would appear and bite her. She demonstrated her capacity to test reality by putting her hand in the toilet, and when "Jaws" did not appear, she stopped being afraid.)

A young adolescent described by E. R. Geleerd (1958) used her mother to integrate her reality testing. When, during a visit, the mother expressed grief over seeing her daughter full of ideas of reference, such as her strong feeling that her friends were wishing her dead, the girl corrected these ideas as she noticed her mother's sadness in relation to her.

SENSE OF SELF

As noted, borderline children do not convey a distinct sense of me-ness. The disturbances in the sense of self indicate certain developmental fixations or regression points. They may perceive themselves as different, without continuity, from one situation to the next. They fail to anticipate gratification or even to show it, nor do they evidence enjoyment in their activities, especially in play. Also missing is an age-appropriate capacity for realistic self-esteem or mastery. Overall, the feeling tone is one of apathy, anhedonia, and worthlessness, and their chronic depression is often compounded by parental and peer rejection as well as by academic problems.

Borderline PD children lack the capacity to internalize gratification because they have not achieved object-constancy—that is, the integration of a representation of a good enough mother. Instead, there is a disturbed sense of self, with distrust and fear of disintegration (Geleerd 1958; Mahler et al. 1949). The bodily self is included here, too (viz., the anxiety and fear of annihilation revealed in the fantasy of a 7-year-old borderline child in analysis, who wanted to play football, but only under certain conditions. He would wear an inflatable outfit, which would expand with air so as practically to invade the whole field. Thus, he would be well-protected, and anybody who bumped against him would only hit him on the surface).

Other experiences also reflect the child's unstable self-concept and difficulties in the separation/individuation process. She may feel that she cannot survive without the other, as if they were hooked, so mother or "another" has to stand by on an ongoing basis, always there. The borderline PD youngster may feel like the toddler whose mother is permanently out of the room, to paraphrase E. C. M. Frijling-Schreuder (1969). Also, the child may indicate that he is beyond danger and needs nobody. Yet on different occasions he will try to control someone else or submit entirely to another's control in order to gain some sense of self (P. Kernberg 1983). As R. Ekstein and S. Friedman (1967) have described, borderline PD children may reverse self and object, much as adult borderline patients do. Accordingly, in treatment they may take on the therapist's role and assign to the therapist the role of patient—sometimes so vividly that the therapist literally feels like the patient.

The fantasy systems articulated below express ways in which the border-line children and adolescent may experience the self, corresponding to M. S. Mahler's phases of separation/individuation.

> I am hooked to my mother, and therefore she cannot survive without me or I without her (Figure IVb)—in the differentiation stage. (This formulation contrasts with the symbiotic vision characteristic of psychosis in which self and object are fused with no boundaries—"I and mother are one" [Figure IVa].)
> I carry mother all around, and I don't need her (Figure IVc)—in the early practicing subphase.
> Mother is inside and part of me for a while. If she is not around, I may cease to exist—lose her inside of me—and therefore I need her around to refuel (Figure IVd)—in the practicing phase proper.

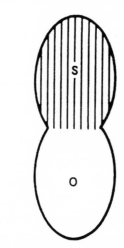

FIGURE IVa   Symbiotic Phase

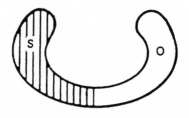

FIGURE IVb   Early differentiation

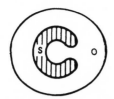

FIGURE IVc   Early practicing

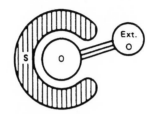

FIGURE IVd   Practicing proper

Mother is not part of me, or I am not part of mother, but instead she is under my control, or I am under her control (Figure IVe)—in the rapprochement phase.

What appears descriptively as fear of merging may, in our opinion, have a
variety of structural implications different from those of the truly symbiotic
psychosis, where self and object dissolve into each other and feel like one. In
borderline cases, fears and wishes of merging *preserve* the distinction between self- and object-images, primitive as these may be. Therefore, we propose that borderline conditions may stem not only from the rapprochement
crisis, but also from fixations or regressions to the earlier differentiation or
practicing phases of the separation/individuation process.

Structurally, self- and object-images are differentiated from each other, but
the relationship varies according to the substage of the separation/individ-
uation process in question. In the early differentiation subphase, self- and
object-image may still have a common partial core (Figure IVa). In the next
stage, the early practicing subphase, we have a self surrounded by the object-image (Figure IVb). The practicing phase proper could be represented as
a self-image having introjected the object-image (Figure IVc); because of the
increased capacity to recognize the reality of separateness, there is a need for

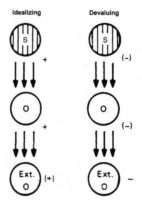

FIGURE IVe   Rapprochement. Left, shadowing. Right, coercion

S = self-image
O = object-image
Ext. O = external object
Reprinted with modifications from: Kernberg, P. F. (1979), Psychoana-
lytic profile of the borderline adolescent. In: S. C. Feinstein, P. L. Gio-
vacchini (eds.). *Adolescent Psychiatry Development and Clinical Studies,
Volume VII.* Chicago: University of Chicago Press, pp. 234–256.

the external object to reinforce or refuel the introjected object image. Last,
the wish for, and the fear of, merging in the rapprochement subphase really
means the need to control or coerce the external object or to be controlled
and coerced by the external object, with increased need for the external object's presence to reinforce and protect the frail stability of achieved self- and
object-differentiation in the absence of object constancy (Figure IVd). The
borderline patient's attempts to achieve a sense of identity and autonomous
functioning is forever unattainable.

Problems in the rapprochement crisis in the separation/individuation
process lead to the persistence of splitting, a weakening mechanism of defense. Splitting in turn interferes with the integration of good and bad images in order to protect the child from anxiety and rage. This seems to be one
of the most prevalent theories about borderline conditions (Mahler et al.
1977). O. Kernberg (1975) has postulated the role of oral aggression leading
to an experience of intense frustration and intense aggression.

Splitting itself may also be caused by constitutional defects that interfere
with the normal mode of integrating perceptions and self- and object-representations, such as attention deficits or other brain dysfunction, or by con-

stitutionally determined lack of anxiety tolerance and excessive aggressive drive—of which the latter factors are not very easily differentiated from pathological parent/child interaction.

PLAY

Borderline children do not play normally or age-appropriately, and they are addicted to pretend play (Weil 1953). Their play has a compulsive, static quality, with little evidence of enjoyment, resolution of conflict, or elaboration of fantasy. According to J. Bemporad and colleagues (1982), these youngsters "can't control their thinking so that they move from neutral themes rapidly into themes of mutilation or death." Games may be tonelessly repeated, or the child may enter into an elementary fantasy play more typical of much younger children, playing at eating or at flying and falling. The incidence of play disruption is higher than in neurotic children. Aggressive and sexual impulses infiltrate the play so that intense anxiety follows; the child is unable to continue playing because the margin between play and the direct expression of drive—the space of make-believe—has collapsed.

EGO FUNCTIONS

SPECIFIC FUNCTIONS

Cognitive deficits affecting attention, spatial orientation, memory, verbal abilities, or such other physical deficiencies as deafness or blindness make children more prone to develop problems of separation/individuation and hence to be at high risk for the development of borderline conditions. In fact, in some adolescent and adult borderline populations, there is increasing evidence of ADHD, other brain dysfunctions, and/or physical deficiencies (Hartocollis 1968).

In relation to motor functions, Weil (1953) has described poor patterning in development, including erratic eating and cleaning habits. Rosenfeld and Sprince (1963) cite unusual movement postures and hyperactivity. For example, a 9-year-old patient diagnosed as having a schizoid personality with borderline features had a very unsteady gait and was so hyperactive that he literally fell from his chair during the initial diagnostic interview. He often bumped into things, and objects accidentally fell from his hands. There was no sign of organicity in the neurological examination, and indeed, his lack of coordination was resolved as he realized that his motor style reflected his identification with his father, who had the same pattern of movements. Borderline adolescents may also have awkward gaits and movements; they may not be as reversible as those of younger ages.

In terms of perception, borderline youngsters are capable of and prone to visual and auditory hallucinations; an important differential diagnosis should be made with the developmentally normal imaginary companion (Nagera 1969). In children, such hallucinations are determined by partial regression without the ominous implications of psychosis that inform adolescents' hallucinations. Many borderline children hear voices inciting them to jump out of the window or reproaching them, or they hear dead people calling them. These hallucinations disappear when anxieties lessen and the child is in a more supportive environment.

According to Coren and Saldinger (1967), the conditions for development of hallucinations in children in general are intense affect, usually aggression; lack of an outlet for this affect; incomplete ego development; poor parental models for reality testing; conflict-laden cathexis of the auditory or visual sphere; a drowsy or tired state; or a traumatic real event that acutely undermines reality testing because it mirrors the child's internal conflict. In borderline children, aggression, incomplete ego development, and poor parental models for reality testing are heavily weighted factors.

No author describes the presence of delusions in borderline adolescents other than in schizophrenia or other adolescent psychosis; borderline conditions are thus differentiated from schizophrenic reactions.

As to reality testing, we agree that there is always contact with reality; although we see no delusions in children, we do concur with E. R. Geleerd (1958) that "their reality testing can be short." The child requires the presence of the object to maintain his sense of reality. In cases of stress, the sense of reality fails, as does reality testing (Pine 1974). Refusal to accept the reality principle makes adaptation to reality inadequate. Although no diagnostic technique has been systemized to assess reality testing in children, the capacity is evaluated through the incidence of play disruption and in terms of the patient's ability to leave her play and come back to everyday life upon termination of the session.

O. Kernberg's (1978) Structural Diagnostic Examination for Adolescents does systematically assess the teenage patient's capacity to test reality in the here-and-now situation. The patient is asked either to evaluate his own behavior and the behavior of the interviewer or to empathize with the different perception that the interviewer may have about his productions. The capacity to empathize with the interviewer's perspective, to at least recognize some social norms with which one may or may not comply, differentiates borderline conditions from schizophrenia (where this capacity does not exist).

NONSPECIFIC FUNCTIONS

The permanent instability of the level of integration of the child and adolescent make these youngsters look well put together at one moment; at the next, falling apart. Likewise, they may appear willing to adhere to rules set for them, only to disavow them impulsively at any moment. Thus their sense of conscience is also brittle.

Nonspecific ego deficits characteristic of the borderline personality are lack of impulse control, low frustration tolerance, low anxiety tolerance, and, we would add, low depression tolerance.

There is also a weakness in the capacity for sublimation so that borderline PD children generally function below their academic potential, even in the absence of learning disabilities. (Indeed, whereas both the child and adolescent can be excellent students, the borderline child does not live up to his potential in graduate school [Gunderson 1977] and usually settles for work actually below his capacities at the professional or career level.)

The aforementioned deficits are common to both children and adolescents, and lack of impulse control in particular seems to be a hallmark of borderline function. Importantly, the lack of control of the different levels of ego organization may not necessarily represent a lack of capacity to exercise control; rather, it may be deployed defensively to bring about different ego states to forestall anxiety.

COPING AND DEFENSE MECHANISMS

As just stated, borderline children suffer from poor tolerance for anxiety, frustration, and depression. They fail to engage in goal-directed activities, and even if their perceptual, motor, and intellectual capacities are intact, they do not use them creatively or effectively. Overall, then, there is a deficit in adaptation (Leichtman and Nathan 1983).

Their defenses have a rigid, yet tenuous, quality. Borderline PD children resort to primitive defenses, such as projective identification, splitting, withdrawal into fantasy, denial, primitive idealization, omnipotent control, and regression in the form of devaluation. They may experience brief psychotic episodes related to stress, with paranoid symptoms, derealization, dissociation, and suicide attempts, lasting a few hours to a day or two.

It is vital to distinguish brittle defenses or failure of defenses from a lack of psychological differentiation and structure. Clinical experience suggests that structured, although primitive, forms of defense *are* present in borderline states. A problem is that these defense mechanisms may in themselves be ego-weakening (O. Kernberg 1975); they should not be confused with the real ego deficits borderline children may also have. The differential diagnosis depends on the child's ability to reconstitute at a higher level when these defense mechanisms are clarified and verbalized in the clinical interaction (P. Kernberg 1988).

The concept of failure in defense or brittle defense is based on the assumption that prior to repression and the classical mechanisms of defense, there is a lack of differentiation and structure. Primitive forms of denial, idealization, devaluation, and projection become apparent as one observes the patient in individual treatment or in the family context.

Weil (1953) discusses the presence of an ineffective type of "faulty repression," and Ekstein and Wallerstein (1954) cite the aggression easily elicited by frustration, which causes abrupt leaps in the use of different levels of defense mechanisms and occurs in the absence of gross external stimuli. These descriptions of defense mechanisms closely overlap with O. Kernberg's (1975) statement that repression is not the main mechanism of defense in borderline conditions but that, rather, splitting is, with all the accompanying mechanisms of omnipotence, primitive forms of projections and denial.

PSYCHOLOGICAL TESTING

A common battery for psychological assessment includes the Weschler Intelligence Scale for Children (Revised) (WISC-III); Wide Range Achievement Test; Benton Visual Memory Test; Draw-a-Person; Illinois Test of Psycholinguistic Abilities; Raven Progressive Matrices; Thematic Apperception Test (TAT); Rorschach and Neuropsychological Screening Tasks (time-orientation, sequencing, laterality, motor functioning, visual-motor functioning, sensory processing, memory functioning, and general academic functioning).

In general, borderline PD patients perform better in structured tests, such as the Wechsler Adult Intelligence Scale or WISC-R, than in relatively unstructured tests like the Rorschach. Answers on unstructured tests reveal a protocol so disturbed as to suggest that they were given by two different people. In spite of the inaccuracies in perception, faulty reasoning, and poor control, the disturbances are mostly ego-syntonic (Exner and Weiner 1982).

Chris was a 7-year-old boy referred for personality testing by a neuropsychologist who felt cognitive factors were not responsible for his academic difficulties. His Rorschach responses included several of poor form level and one fabulized combination. There were many eyes in several of his Rorschach responses, suggesting a paranoid orientation. His other responses further raised the question of delusional thinking, problems in reality testing, and immature and/or regressive functioning. The presence of confabulations indicated that his judgment could be poor resulting from inferential leaps he might make based on partial information.

Therefore, following the Rorschach Test, he was asked, simply, "tell me about your imagination." He understood the concept and the difference between imagination and reality. He described imagining monsters in his backyard with his friend, which sounded playful. He also imagined monsters when alone, specifically conceiving shadows as monsters at night that would eat him up: "some look like Dracula, and I'm afraid they'll bite me and turn me into another Dracula." He said that even though he thinks a lot about monsters, he does not think they are real. When asked about auditory hallucinations, Chris identified phenomena outside of him: "The voices are all around . . . sometimes like they're going to attack or something like that." He said he thought this part was real, not his imagination, and that he had a procedure to control the voices: turning his head to one side could make the voices start over again; turning his head another way stopped them. He sometimes turned his head the wrong way and by mistake sent the voices back to the "beginning," as if they were a record. He said he had not told anyone about this, including his parents and his therapist, but he did want the examiner to tell them, and he wanted help "because when that happens it feels like I'm not a normal person." He himself told his parents about it after this session.

Chris was not able to use his excellent intellect (e.g., scaled score of 18 on the WISC-R Similarities subtest) to organize the world when a great deal of affective stimulation occurred quickly with little structure; he could do so, however, with more structure, as reflected in his fine understanding of social causality on the WISC-R (Picture Arrangement = 14). Thus, Card II, the first presentation of color on the Rorschach Test, elicited a response using very little form, indicating the disruptive effect that emotion and interpersonal demands can have on him ("It's like an explosion, a big explosion. There's the fire, and here's the smoke").The response reflected Chris's struggle to develop an autonomous, integrated sense of self against countervailing forces in his family (Card I: "Two things pulling apart an ant, two people" . . . "It's not coming apart yet; they're trying to pull it apart"), but the tension, inadequacy, and hopelessness he may have felt as the small, struggling ant was reflected in his third response to Card I ("A plane split in half"). His response to the last Rorschach card offered a code to the theme of autonomy and the establishment of boundaries and a sense of self (Card X: "Cells . . . they're, like, enlarged. Cells don't have any shape. If it's an animal cell with no cell wall, it doesn't have any shape, and this doesn't have any shape . . . and this looks like a microscope with an eyepiece and knobs").

The aggression described by his parents and by him (he liked fighting with his brother, which was what he would miss if his brother died) may serve both as a way of creating contact with others and getting them to react. Their reaction would provide a basis for his affirmation of self-boundaries with parents who describe themselves as emotionally absent and avoidant of direction and limit setting.

Adam, a 10-year-old like Chris, has a strong reaction to the first appearance of color on Card II ("Looks like a bloody face"), but Adam shows greater use of form, implying greater intellectual control and resources. Indeed, he continues on Card II ("two people giving each other a high five") and on Card III ("two people playing the drum") with excellent, integrative responses showing good boundaries and representation of others. However, his ambivalence and split view of others, more characteristic of much younger children, was readily apparent in his second response to Card II ("two people pulling out the eyes of an alien").

The malevolence in this Rorschach image was reflected in a more passive manner on the TAT, where the maternal neglect and hostility he described is expressed (Card V: "Looks like the mother's looking into the room. There is no story because there's nothing happening." Then, "This looks like a kid's head," referring to a vase in the picture on a table in a scene in which a woman is looking into a room through a partially opened door. As to the next, "Nothing to tell a story about. She looks into the room and sees the kid's head on a table, I don't know, a funeral . . . she's sorry she ever left the kid alone. Otherwise he wouldn't be dead. He got on the table, fell off, and killed himself. Trying to get to the cookie jar"). It was as if the first Rorschach image was completed and he, in taking it apart, exposed the child's internalization of the mother's wish to be rid of him and not be bothered by having children to take care of. His perception here shows an isolated but meaningful break with reality. His story also reflects themes about loss, separation, neediness, and rejection, which are often seen in the stories of borderline children, including those presented here.

Eleven-year-old Carl's overall intellectual level was in the superior range, with his verbal score being nonsignificantly higher than his performance score. His intelligence test responses included intrusive material in a manner not seen with Adam or Chris. For example, he manipulated the pieces of the "girl" in an unusual way after he completed this WISC-R Object Assemble item. When asked what was happening, he said he was "killing her."

His Rorschach Test begins by demonstrating his anxiety and bodily concerns (Card I, first response: "A spider missing two legs"), later followed by an attempt at compensation (Card I, third response: "A bat with four extra wings"). When he first saw affectivity stimulating material with Card II, he responded with great emotion—"Oh boy, oh boy, oh boy"—but tried to use denial and reacted in a very passive, externalizing way ("That doesn't really show me anything"). After a relatively long latency, he responded (Card II, first response: "An alien space ship with blood bombs firing"; second response: "An engine that runs on blood"), with the less modulated aggressive affect dominating his perception; form was secondary. He as much as recognized this with his comment, "an alien space ship can be any shape."

Card III did not lead to the conventional response of a person. Instead, Carl portrayed a malevolent object, and the sequence indicated his fear of the bad object (mother) that enhances itself by devouring others. There was a paranoid, almost delusional quality to the fear. His reality testing became poor, and the symbolic use of achromatic color was suggestive of the disordered thinking associated with depressed mood (Card III: "A weird bug with very sharp teeth and a heart that shows with visible markings so nobody can get it, and it looks like it is pulling two seahorses in with it. I have quite an imagination!" "A heart, which should be painted black . . . because bugs are mean . . . because bugs should have black hearts if they're mean"). His comments about his "imagination" and being "sick" suggested that thoughts such as these made him afraid that he was crazy. He recovered, however, and gave conventional, intelligible, popular responses to Cards IV and V.

In both structured and unstructured tests, borderline children show fluidity of associations, peculiar logic, and flights into fantasy. M. Engel (1963) emphasized the particular intense involvement that borderline children develop with the examiner. Engel adds that in contrast to psychotic children, borderline children are able to portray their massive anxiety in realistic fantasies and stories. According to M. Leichtman and S. Shapiro (1980b), these children have no expectation of themselves and no motivation to give a right answer. There is a lack of phase-dominance in terms of drives, and in the Rorschach Test, one often observes inanimate movement responses and sexualization of responses as counterphobic maneuvers. Fear of the inkblots and anxiety reactions may be extreme, with concerns about survival, separation, and destruction; anxiety easily escalates to panic. In terms of thought disorder, one sometimes encounters strange associations and preservations with little tendency to reality adherence. There is also a quality of playing "crazy" when people appear.

Object-representations within the Rorschach Test seem to be unrealistic and unidimensional. The few human percepts tend to split into all good and bad figures (grandiose/impotent, idealized/malevolent). One sees a regressive experience of merger, or rather partial merger, in the sense of one person being attached to another. Leichtman and Shapiro (1980b), for instance, report two-headed people, Siamese twins, two Martians fused together, two elephants joined together at the tail, or two women chanting in unison. Also apparent are themes of loss, separation, and abandonment with helplessness and primitive aggression. The tenuous sense of identity is illustrated by body-image distortions showing a strong identification with extraterrestrial beings, anxiety about disappearance, and visions of people about to explode.

A. D. Blotcky (1984) offered a practical application of the Rorschach tests in anticipation of transference developments of borderline adolescents, specifically through their use of primitive idealization and devaluation. Patients frequently cite paired figures with negative valences or behaviors—two ugly men or women, two monsters, two people or animals stuck together or hating each other—rather than positive images (two really happy heroes, two great human giants, two angels in love).

Only recently, the Minnesota Multiphasic Personality Inventory has been studied in relation to borderline PD. We introduce it as an independent validator of borderline PD diagnosis in adolescents to be used in conjunction with other tests and not by itself. R. P. Archer and colleagues (1985) studied 146 consecutively admitted adolescents between 12 and 18 years of age—82 percent white, 11 percent black, 7 percent other ethnic backgrounds—from lower- to middle-socioeconomic class. They were selected according to *DSM-III* diagnostic criteria, applying norm conversions for the MMPI in adolescent populations.

Adolescents with borderline PD had significantly higher MMPI mean scores on five scales—(Hs) Hypochondriasis, (D) Depression, (Sc) Schizophrenia, (MF) Masculinity-Femininity, and (Pd) Psychopathic Deviate—than those in the comparison groups, who were adolescents with conduct disorders, dysthymic disorders, and other PDs. The combination of the MMPI scales (MF, D, Pa, Pd, Pt, K, and Sc)* accounted for 59 percent of the variance between borderline PD and the control group.

The similarity of MMPI scenes found in adolescents and adults with PDs points to the congruence of the clinical symptomatology of these two age groups.

ETIOLOGY

BIOLOGICAL AND GENETIC FACTORS

There is increasing evidence of neurological disturbances, probably due to the high incidence of abuse: sexual, physical, and verbal. D. L. Gardner and colleagues (1987) found a significantly higher incidence of soft neurological signs that suggests abnormal neurological development or disturbances in neurological organization of function. M. H. Teicher and colleagues (1994) and Van der Kolk and Greenberg (1987) have linked childhood abuse to a kindling of the limbic system that codetermines the typical symptoms of these patients—affective lability, impulsivity, aggression, and dissociative states, among others. Post and colleagues (1984) have shown how the amigdala connects to aggressive behaviors and how episodic dyscontrol can present excitatory functions through kindling long after the traumatic event.

The differential roles of the right and left hemispheres in the perception of emotions and in language function respectively point toward a neurological basis for dissociation and/or splitting mechanisms (Davidson et al. 1990). Front temporal areas are significantly more affected in the EEG in abused patients than in nonabused patients (Teicher et al. 1994).

---

*Pa denotes Paranoia; Pt denotes Psychasthenia (inability to resist undesirable maladaptive behaviors); K denotes Validity indicator.

The neurobiological model refers to the frequent association of borderline PD with impaired central nervous system functioning. The various deficits affect the child's internal and external world of experience, the construction of the internal representation world (Sandler and Rosenblatt 1962), the internal working scheme of self and others (Bowlby 1969, Stern 1985), and their interpersonal world. These deficits refer to impulsivity, low frustration tolerance, controls over cognition, attention, affect, and integrative functions: They put the child at risk for borderline ego development codetermined by an organic pathway. Substance abuse, alcoholism, and histrionic and sociopathic behaviors are concomitant phenomena in these behaviors.

Andrulonis and colleagues (1980) provided further contributions to understanding a neurobehavioral basis: 53 percent of male patients presented with minimal brain dysfunction or learning disability, as compared with 13.5 percent of female patients.

The "organic" borderline pattern presents an early childhood onset of impulsive acting out, substance abuse, and mild depression. In contrast, the predominantly female "nonorganic" borderlines typically had an adolescent onset of greater depression and a family history of affective disorder.

H. P. Soloff and J. W. Millward (1983) have presented an excellent outline of the developmental hypothesis for borderline PD. Their research compared the developmental histories of borderline patients with those of patients with affective and schizophrenic disorders in an attempt to validate borderline PD as an independent construct. Complications of pregnancy were significantly higher for borderline patients, as were tendencies for prematurity and low birth weight. A continuum of learning difficulties was found, from most severe in schizophrenics to intermediate in borderlines and least severe among depressed patients. Temper tantrums, head banging, and rocking were highly prevalent in borderline patients versus the other two groups, as was a strikingly high use of alcohol and drugs in borderline and schizophrenics, as compared with depressed controls.

Although there is currently evidence for the heritability of personality traits, there is no evidence for the heritability of borderline PD. According to A. A. Dahl (1985), the estimate that 38 percent of borderline patients have a relative with a depressive disorder is probably low; patients and informants tend to underreport when compared to direct examination of the relatives. Moreover, A. W. Loranger and colleagues (1982) have found that the first-degree relatives of borderline patients have a morbidity risk for developing borderline PD nearly 10 times that of the relatives of bipolar and schizophrenic probands. The risk for unipolar depression in borderline PD relatives is similar to the risk for bipolar disorder relatives; there does not seem to be an increased risk for bipolar disorders in relatives of borderline PD probands, however. H. G. Pope and colleagues (1983) also found increased prevalence of borderline PD in first-degree relatives of borderline PD.

The separation hypothesis suggests the important role of separation and loss or the threat of loss through withdrawal of parental affection. The separation/individuation process is affected, producing a developmental arrest characterized by the persistence of primitive defenses and a failure to achieve object constancy.

Soloff and Millward (1983) assessed borderline patients in terms of the intactness of their families: Patients suffered a significantly greater incidence of paternal loss by death or divorce compared with a control group. According to Soloff and Millward, borderline patients showed problems in more areas of developmental separation than the other groups, especially as they grew into adulthood—64 percent borderlines, 37 percent depressed, and 3 percent schizophrenics. This study demonstrates increased separation experiences and increased sensitivity for separation in borderline patients. (Separation here is taken as severance from an important paternal figure.)

FAMILY PSYCHODYNAMICS

One frequently finds pervasive pathological interactions within the families of borderline adolescents (Shapiro et al. 1975) and children. The family situation tends to maintain borderline functioning. There is anxiety about supporting the child's autonomy and a denial of her dependence. Parents may use the child narcissistically, and dyadic relations between the child and each parent predominate. J. Bemporad and colleagues (1982) remarked on the chaotic nature of parent/child interaction, often reflecting abuse, neglect, and bizarre behaviors on the part of the parents, as well as inconsistent care. Ten out of 24 children in Bemporad's sample were physically abused.

D. B. Rinsley (1981) summarized his conception of the developmental arrest that borderlines present in terms of their separation/individuation failure, beginning at the practicing subphase—and, we would add, the differentiation subphase (P. Kernberg 1979)—and reaching its peak during the rapprochement subphase.

Shapiro and colleagues (1975) indicate the pervasiveness of pathological interactions within families of borderline adolescents. In their research on hospitalized borderline adolescents receiving family therapy, they cite the abundant use of projective identification in the family setting that, if not necessarily causal, contributes to maintaining borderline functioning. Each member of the family sees himself as "strong and autonomous," without dependent needs, whereas the designated child is perceived as weak, vulnerable and demanding, and totally dependent. Independence and separation from family are taken as devaluation of family values, or dependency is experienced as an overwhelming and dangerous burden on the family. The parents unconsciously perceive the child's independent moves as hostile rejections of her needs for nurturing and support as demands.

Shapiro and colleagues (1975) also noted that primitive defenses, such as splitting, good/bad, and projective identification, operate equally at the level of the family group. The child enacts the role of parent, and the parent enacts the role of child. The child has to modify his objective experience in accordance with these projections. Splitting and projective identification impairs the child's ego formation: The child is unable to tolerate the parent's or his own anxiety.

A 17-year-old was hospitalized two weeks for destructive behavior after his own mother was hospitalized for a suicide attempt. In the preceding months, he had wanted to work and was successful in finding employment on a newspaper. His mother, a chronically depressed woman, became so panicky about his moving out of the home and being more independent that she told him that she would not be around anymore and attempted to commit suicide. After her hospitalization, he became upset and withdrawn, and for two weeks stayed home, doing nothing. Finally, he had an abrupt outburst of temper, breaking chairs and furniture, and forcing his father, a passive and withdrawn man, to hospitalize him. Once in the hospital, however, he reorganized, feeling relieved to be away from the family. In those patients where endowment is adequate, the role of the family, and specifically the mother, in the separation/individuation phase seems to be crucial.

Other forms of pathological communication between the family members have been described (Rinsley 1981), including narcissistic use of the child, inconsistency, dominant intrusive behavior, and depersonification of the child who is treated as an object to soothe mother's anxieties and not as a subject in her own right. The mother exerts such control over the child that she submits to the cruel object in the hope of eventually triumphing and obtaining love. Extreme forms of masochistic surrender to the idealized mother may stem from this mechanism, which interferes with the expression of aggression and maintains splitting, thus fostering the formation of borderline personality organization.

Soloff and Millward's (1983) findings illustrated that among borderline patients' families, the overall pattern is one of severe pathology, with intrusive controlling mothers, distant or hostile fathers, and conflictual marital relationships. Fathers of borderline patients contribute to the risk of borderline PD in their offspring either by being passive and/or noninvolved or through hostile rejection, a pattern commonly observed in father/son or mother/daughter relationships. We add another constellation, whereby the mother is in the role of the one parent whereas the father's place is to be one more sibling among the children.

How stable is the diagnosis of borderline PD over time? The predictive validity of the diagnosis is relatively low. Fifty percent of the borderlines followed up by T. H. McGlashan (1983) retained their original diagnosis, 20 percent got a diagnosis of schizophrenia or schizoaffective disorder, and only a few had developed major affective disorders.

Borderline PD overlaps with hysterical, antisocial, or narcissistic PDs, which points to the usefulness of a personality organization concept (O. Kernberg 1975). Schizotypal personality can be considered a prepsychotic PD, a stable one evolving into schizophrenia or a residual state of schizophrenia. Prospective studies are needed to study this problem.

Suicide attempts in borderlines are less than 10 percent, no different from that found in affective psychosis and schizophrenia. Substance abuse is more common in borderline PDs and indicates a worse outcome.

PROGNOSIS

In their four- to seven-year follow-up study, H. G. Pope and colleagues showed that 26 percent of their patients had good global outcome, and 48 percent had poor global outcome. In contrast, T. H. McGlashan's study, which is a longer follow-up study (15 years), indicates that the borderline PD group did significantly better than Pope's groups, and that depression makes the outcome somewhat worse rather than better, as Pope indicated in his study.

OBJECT-RELATIONS

RELATIONSHIP TO MATERNAL REPRESENTATION

The borderline child's relationship to the mother is characterized either by primitive idealization of the object, with the patient sharing in what is perceived as the object's goodness and power, or attribution of extreme meanness to the mother and at times devaluation (Geleerd 1958, Mahler 1977, Weil 1953, Rosenfeld and Sprince 1963). Mother is perceived as controlling or invasive. As described by E. R. Shapiro and colleagues (1975) in research on families of borderline adolescents, the parents are perceived as all good or all bad, according to the need to split and to differentiate the good mother of separation from the bad mother of separation. Splitting features prominently in the borderline child's object-relations.

The child tends to relate either to mother (to the exclusion of father) or to father (to the exclusion of mother). There is an inability to relate to the parents as a couple. There is also an inability to deal with sibling rivalry and envy, often with expressions of intense hostility against siblings and even outright sibling abuse.

Clinical observation suggests that borderline children do not have transitional objects as a rule; when they do, the objects acquire a bizarre quality. The existence of a transitional object presupposes some internalization of a positive object relation with the mother in order that the child can reproduce it in an intermediate world of experience. The borderline child has not developed a positive sense of self in relation to a positive object, however, so it is not surprising that he lacks a transitional object at the appropriate age (8 to 24 months) or of the usual quality (such as a soft toy). Instead, borderline PD youngsters tend to cling directly to their mothers, possibly searching for symbiotic-like experiences or positive feelings—or else they may represent their relationship to the bad mother by attaching themselves to a mechanical object. (One child, for instance, used a robot as a transitional object, taking it with him wherever he went.) Finally, if a borderline child does adopt a transitional object, it is apt to portray a part of the child's self (e.g., a hat) rather than to reflect the gestalt of the experience with mother (say, by means of texture or smell).

FRIENDSHIPS AND PEER RELATIONSHIPS

The defects of borderline children's internal object-relations can be seen in their use of others as part-objects or outright self-objects. Other people's individual characteristics are completely missed; indeed, the borderline PD patient lives in a world where the other is only a vehicle for her own projections—a "thing" to be leaned upon, controlled, idealized, or devalued. Such interactions are poignantly expressed in the child's relationships to peers, which fluctuate from apparent sociability to withdrawal. Variously indiscriminate and too possessive, 90 percent of borderline children have poor peer relations (Bentivegna et al. 1985). In spite of having social skills, they seem unable to maintain friendships, ending in a chronic sense of isolation.

AFFECTS

Various authors working with children (Pine 1974, Rosenfeld and Sprince 1963, Geleerd 1958) agree that the borderline child's anxiety is intense and free-floating. It is an anxiety of total loss, disaster, and annihilation, with a traumatic quality quite different from the signal anxiety of neurotic patients.

As M. S. Mahler and colleagues observed in 1949, rage with proneness to tantrums is prevalent. Aggression may reach dangerous levels, as in poking a pencil in the eye of a schoolmate, throwing a baby brother against the wall, or seriously threatening to jump out of the window.

Affects are sudden, abrupt (see Pine 1974, Rosenfeld and Sprince 1963), and of an all-or-nothing quality, with direct discharge or no discharge at all. One sees immaturity and wide mood swings. We can understand the latter as derivatives of the mood swings in the separation/individuation process—that is, elation in the practicing subphases and depressive moods alternating with a sense of omnipotence in the rapprochement crisis. Thus, an angry coercive attitude and a hypomanic-like elation can be considered as the affective counterpart of the main fixation point of borderline children's psychopathology—the separation/individuation subphases, especially the rapprochement crisis. R. Grinker et al. (1968) refers to similar mood swings in adult borderline patients.

There appears to be a lack of guilt, concern, assessment in depth of others, commitment to a set of values (cultural and artistic), and no possibility of nonexploitative relationships. Missing also are the affect-modulated derivatives of a synthesis of positive and negative self- and object-representations into an integrated concept—namely, what M. S. Mahler (1975) has described as the state of being on the way to object constancy.

Similar affective qualities are described in borderline adolescents: intense anger, demandingness (an expression of coercion), exploitative behavior, and lack of social tact. Grinker (1968) described mood swings, depression with hostile rage reactions, and self-destructiveness or detached, mute behavior associated with a passive show of anger. This latter characteristic coincides with E. R. Geleerd's (1958) observation that there is either aggression or no direct expression of aggression at all. Like borderline children, who lack the capacity to anticipate and even experience enjoyment and pleasure (as their virtual inability to use play for these purposes reveals), borderline adolescents are unable to experience true satisfaction and pleasure.

The high incidence of associated depression in these patients deserves attention. In adults, there is increasing evidence of a strong association between borderline personality organization and major affective disorders, as if the major affective disorder preserved and maintained borderline personality organization; here, genetic aspects are important (Pope et al. 1983). The child's sense of worthlessness and helplessness is compounded by difficulties interacting with others: He does not derive gratification from mutuality and reciprocity in maternal, paternal, or peer relations. To the contrary, he is rejected and disliked for his primitive ways of relating.

Additionally, borderline children are persecuted by terrifying superego forerunners, as in the case of the girl who was afraid of being eaten up by "Jaws." The incapacity to derive pleasure from play or to use it to neutralize frustration and aggression adds to their helplessness, leading to chronic depressive affect. Lastly, the frequent coexistence of organicity makes for difficulties in learning and social interaction, again compounding their inability to cope and further worsening depression. This multidetermined depression combines with impulsivity (rooted either in the borderline personality organization itself or in organicity) so that suicide attempts are a frequent cause of hospitalization (Pfeffer 1982). (A tendency to react severely to loss, poorly controlled anger, and self-defeating impulsivity correlate with suicide attempts in borderline adolescents, Crumley 1981.)

SUPEREGO INTEGRATION

There is a unanimous sense that early developmental experiences have an impact on superego formation (Pine 1974, Rosenfeld and Sprince 1963). Superego development, because of the splitting and the lack of synthetic function of the ego, remains at the level of introjects, easily projected onto external objects—hence, the paranoid potential of borderline PD patients. (The adolescent borderline frequently produces micropsychotic transferences with a paranoid flavor.) The use of primitive defenses, particularly splitting and projective identification denial, relates to their difficulties in assuming responsibility for their actions, in other words, their shifting level of superego functioning.

FANTASIES

E. R. Geleerd (1958) and R. Ekstein and S. Friedman (1967) have discussed the fantasy life of the borderline child. No relinquishment of omnipotent fantasy occurs. The fantasies come from all levels of psychosexual development and are sexual as well as aggressive. The child is easily made anxious and becomes overwhelmed by these fantasies. For example, a 7-year-old patient was afraid to light matches because, if he did, fire would invade the entire street and destroy New York City, the United States, and the world, and would only "stop short of the north and south poles where there are 7, no, 700 feet of ice." He would never play with matches for sure. According to Ekstein and Friedman, a feeling of external danger usually goes along with fantasies; consequently, they are not sources of much gratification.

Typical in regressed ego states are fears of separation and abandonment, bodily disintegration, and distortion of body image. A patient aged 6, for example, swallowed his baby teeth as his permanent teeth replaced them. Fantasies connected with oedipal levels may mask problems deriving from earlier stages of development.

Masturbatory fantasies with oedipal components, combined with fantasies of aggression and fantasies of other perverse activities permeated with aggression, are common in both children and adolescents. There is no clearcut period of latency. Similarly, compulsive masturbation with perverse fantasies is frequent. One borderline child, for example, had masturbatory fantasies that included the idea of flooding the world with urine. He pictured his mother's dying under his father's beatings. An adolescent patient dreamed she had intercourse with a blade that would cut her so badly she might die.

CHARACTERISTICS OF THE OEDIPAL SITUATION

The borderline child, as well as the adolescent, experiences oedipal situations that are distorted by the weight of the unresolved difficulties in the separation/individuation stages—issues of agency versus differentiation versus merging and autonomy versus coercive control. The phallic stage is unstable. As the inability to separate from the mother enhances incestuous ties, the boy has increased problems of disidentification with the mother and is predisposed to sexual disturbance. In the borderline child or adolescent, fear of annihilation by maternal abandonment increases the difficulty of separating to invest in others. The individual has not achieved the autonomy conferred by self-constancy and object-constancy. Hence the occurrence of being alone, which is evidenced in problems with peers and in the adolescent, heterosexual relations characterized by extreme forms of sadistic control of the partner or by altruistic surrender or shadowing.

TREATMENT

Psychodynamic Therapy

Psychodynamic therapy aiming at symptomatic improvement but also at a resumption of development and personality integration must address the following issues:

Aberrant development versus developmental arrest. It seems to be more true to the picture one sees in borderline children to conceptualize an aberrant development course with accrual of distortions in practically every aspect of the personality than to postulate arrest per se. It is not that development has not proceeded but that it has followed a skewed course. This distinction has ramifications for the treatment approach. With most borderline children, it would be a mistake to base the therapy only on supportive interventions or environmental manipulations. Instead, it is necessary to undo and resolve extreme character pathology and conflict configurations.

Is ego organization inherently unstable? Some authors have described the instability of the ego in borderline patients as a fluid ego organization (Ekstein and Wallerstein 1954). In our experience, however, the shifting ego states correspond to organized self- and object-representations that are activated for defensive purposes and for primary and secondary gains, to deal with frustration or anxiety. The more typical coping mechanisms of neurosis, such as affiliation, humor, sublimation, and suppression, are not so readily observed among borderlines. Instead, one finds coercion, shadowing, withdrawal, regression, or direct temper outbursts, and each of these corresponds to the activation of different self- and object-representations.

Kenny, an 8-year-old boy, had broken the window of the garage. He had also been stealing pencils from his peers at school. When confronted with this misbehavior, he blamed two or three children in a rather diffuse manner. He was unable to feel any guilt and, instead, seemed only fleetingly embarrassed; indeed, he was furious about even being confronted. When told by his mother that he would not be allowed any Halloween candy, he denied that the punishment was fair and pretended to be in a very good mood. At first, he sucked his thumb and appeared to try to control his reaction in that way. Soon thereafter he assumed a flippant attitude and declared that he was going to get candy anyhow; in fact, the school bus driver had already given him some. In the next half-hour, a variety of expressive reactions ensued, including temper outbursts, projection, coercive behavior with the mother, and throwing an object at the therapist. Kenny tried to deal with the situation inefficiently through mechanisms of denial, regression, omnipotent control, and discharge into action. These shifting behaviors did not necessarily arise out of any intrinsic instability of his ego states but corresponded to a structured repertoire of maladaptive defense maneuvers.

The question of ego weakness. An important consideration in treatment, this global concept needs to be spelled out in its particulars. After all, the ego is a system containing many functions, only one of which is object relations. Moreover, ego weakness in itself can be used for defensive purposes, adding most crucial leverage in interpretative work with these patients. The very expectations of the therapist who postulates an irreversible ego defect rather than a special form of defense by the ego may make the child's unreachability by therapeutic interaction a self-fulfilling prophecy.

Do borderline conditions blend with psychotic conditions? An understanding of this question is crucial for the conduct of psychotherapy. Certainly, borderline children may have brief psychotic episodes related to stress, with paranoid symptoms, depersonalization, derealization, dissociation, and suicide attempts. We must look at the distinguishing nature of defenses and anxieties in the psychotic patient and at his lack of differentiation between self and object.

Typical psychotic defenses include the most primitive forms of projection, fragmentation, and somatization, such as extreme hypochondriasis, animation of inanimate objects, deanimation of animate objects, formation of bizarre objects, delusions, and hallucinations. The anxieties do not entail fears of annihilation so much as fears of falling, losing oneself through dissolving, and total fragmentation. The incapacity to test reality given the supports of clarification and confrontation further delineates psychosis from borderline conditions.

The psychotic patient's regression to a symbiotic state with no boundaries between self and object is another key difference. In contrast, the fusion fantasies of borderline patients, if looked at carefully, contain the various structural implications that outlined in the description of the experience of self. They illustrate failures in the process of separation/individuation and not regression to an undifferentiated self. It is true that there may be transitory states of regression to and fixation at a pathological symbiotic level, but in most cases the borderline patient can rebound to the differentiation between self and object in one of the other constellations. These formulations have practical implications in terms of the specific interpretive work with the transference in the here-and-now and also in the understanding of countertransference reactions.

PSYCHOPHARMACOLOGIC TREATMENT

In agreement with T. A. Petti (1981), psychopharmacologic agents should be used for target symptoms that interfere with the child's adaptation, but in combination with psychosocial interventions, including psychotherapy in all different modalities—supportive, expressive, cognitive/behavioral, in families, and in groups (Petti 1981).

SEPARATION/INDIVIDUATION DIFFICULTIES

A major goal in the treatment of all borderline children is the resolution of primitive defense patterns by establishing integrated and stable self- and object-representations that facilitate separation (autonomy) and individuation (individuality). The achievement of individuation in turn strengthens the ego. Also important are the attainment of reliable reality testing, facilitation of sublimatory channels, and increased external adjustment. Increasing tolerance for affects, especially anxiety and depression, is another goal.

It is the opinion of many researchers that borderline conditions originate in the separation/individuation phase, in particular in the rapprochement crisis. C. F. Settlage (1977) has underlined the importance of this phase in normal development, and his observations carry implications for understanding and empathizing with the reenactment of its derivatives in the therapeutic interaction. According to Settlage, the mirroring function of the mother entails:

- interest in the child's developing skills;
- attribution of meaning to the child's activities;
- the sharing of power;
- affirmation of the child's expanding sense of self and identity;
- validation of the child's continuing importance to the mother;
- acceptance and management of the child's urges;
- being available when needed; and
- tolerance for regression, as well as for the child's increasing autonomy.

Each of these components of mirroring is also an important function of the therapist as she enables the patient to become aware of early wishes and needs through verbalization.

With the young child, it is possible to handle problems in separating from the mother in a way that differs technically from work with children and adolescents. The task is to resolve the pathological clinging, shadowing, and darting away through joint work with the mother/child pair. More often than not, the pathological attachment to the mother belies an asymmetrical symbiosis-like relationship in which the child may be much more ready to leave the mother than the mother is to leave the child. In working with the mother/child dyad, the therapist systematically explores and brings out the anxiety around individuation—the fears of abandonment and total loss or annihilation. These fears need to be verbalized by both the mother and the child and to be empathized with by the therapist. In this way, the separation/individuation process may be encouraged to proceed toward self- and object-constancy.

A 6-year-old child suffering from an elevator phobia was reluctant to come to the office without his mother. At first, child and mother did not even take off their coats while visiting the therapist. Whenever the child began to play with the therapist, the mother turned her back, yawned, fell asleep, or threatened to leave the room. Frequently they did not even come to the sessions. When the mother's anxiety vis-à-vis the increasing autonomy of the child was clarified, the therapist was perceived as less threatening; eventually, the mother agreed to participate in the sessions.

The child portrayed the various difficulties in separation through his play. In one session, for example, he initially left the therapist outside in the corridor while he and his mother entered the room. Then he allowed the therapist to come into the room. Next, he himself remained outside while the therapist went into the room with his mother. Later on, he put a chair at the threshold of the door and asked the therapist to sit there; then he himself sat there. In the next session, he left the mother alone inside the room, checking on her from time to time. He then went to the elevator, threw some pieces of paper inside, and asked the therapist to step into the elevator while he waited outside. Later, he took elevator rides while the therapist waited outside in the lobby.

Slowly and painfully, both mother and child had a second chance, under the facilitating influence of the therapist, to work through the vicissitudes of separation/individuation.

COMPLICATIONS OF COGNITIVE IMPAIRMENTS

The importance of identifying cognitive impairments when treating borderline children and adolescents cannot be stressed enough: Only by fully defining the problem can the clinician combine all necessary pharmacological, educational, and psychotherapeutic interventions and target appropriate treatments to the symptoms. The patient must be informed about his deficits and learn to accommodate to them. By becoming conscious of and accepting his own limitations, he will be less prone to anxiety and depression and may begin to establish better contact with peers and relevant adults. Working with the parents at the same time to acquaint them with the child's particular difficulties may facilitate their empathic responses. This approach complements quite well the approach used to deal with conflict-based difficulties, namely, working in the here-and-now, interpreting primitive defense mechanisms and negative transference, and providing external structure in cases of acting out.

J. Frosch (1971) and R. R. Greenson (1954) intuitively arrived at the need to work psychotherapeutically not only with these patients' conflicts but also with their understanding of their perceptions and attitudes toward the therapist's interventions. What these two psychoanalysts propose may be a necessary intervention, given that the patients' distorted perceptions of the therapist may be due not only to resistance but also to difficulties in attention and memory, as well as in perceiving social interactions—all hallmarks of a comorbid Attention Deficit Hyperactivity syndrome.

Discontinuities in the perception of the object further enable the use of splitting. For instance, an object may be realistically perceived as different if it is presented from different angles; there may be no capacity to abstract common features. Here the advantage of a psychoanalytically oriented approach lies in the therapist's use of both observation and empathy to elucidate some of the perplexing manifestations of organicity and its possible contributions to borderline functioning.

TECHNICAL CONSIDERATIONS FOR PSYCHOANALYTIC PSYCHOTHERAPY

The treatment approach advocated here is a multimodal one, with attention to both the child and the environment. That is, it may be necessary to work directly with the family to provide a stable and predictable home life and correct pathogenic intrafamilial interactions supporting splitting, projection, and denial.

If these arrangements do not suffice to contain the child's destructive behaviors toward self and others, a day hospital or inpatient setting is indicated—the latter especially in the case of suicidal behavior, runaway behavior, severe school refusal accompanied by regression, anorexia, or lack of minimal family support. Individual psychotherapy with the child can then take place within this structured environment.

The psychoanalytically oriented psychotherapy takes place two or three times a week for a minimum of one or two years. The play materials should be simple and lend themselves to gross motor activities—sponge balls and bowling equipment—or to fantasy play—dolls, soldiers, puppets, superheroes, and rubber monsters of all kinds. Video games are much less useful because they do not promote person-to-person interaction or the elaboration of primitive dissociated fantasies into the fantasy life of play and creativity.

Psychoanalytically oriented psychotherapy with the borderline child involves a number of special considerations for its effectiveness. With clarification of interactions, emphasis belongs on the here-and-now.

It is important that the patient become aware of the actual ongoing interactions with the therapist, who can foster her reality-testing capacity and minimize distortions as well as increase the necessary affective conviction about interpretations. Specifically, the child's perceptions and applications of what she perceives should be continually tested in terms of the reality of the therapist's actions and verbal interventions. Despite the tendency to distort reality through the use of primitive defense mechanisms, one must always remember that the borderline PD patient does, in fact, have the capacity to test reality; in this respect, the therapist acts as an observing ego. Fantasy distortions need to be verbalized and shared to allow for secondary-process reasoning. It is through identification with the therapist's capacity to tolerate these primitive fantasies that the patient comes to feel less anxiety while she develops the capacity to express them through play, dreams, or daydreams.

Clarification of Generational and Sexual Boundaries

If the child is an outpatient, ongoing contact with the parents and/or joint family play sessions to assess and to modify nonverbal interactions are indicated. Family work should aim at supporting and clarifying generational and sexual boundaries and roles. This approach enables the parental couple to include the siblings while maintaining their tie as a couple. We have observed that parents of borderline children more frequently relate to the children as their own siblings or as though they themselves were single; that is, the mother or father relates to the child to the exclusion of the other parent.

Neutralizing Splitting

If the patient is hospitalized, the therapist works alongside the interdisciplinary team, which also receives impressions of the various splitting mechanisms. The therapist integrates and synthesizes direct information from the staff of their different perceptions of the patient and also keeps the team aware of the patient's often subtle projections onto them—thus managing the staff's feelings of anxiousness or hopelessness toward a "cool" or challenging child. Team meetings with the child present to discuss everyday interactions can prove quite useful in working against splitting and other primitive defense mechanisms.

With borderline children, one must recognize that the self-representation, although allowing for the separateness of the object, is not yet integrated. Consider the 7 -year-old boy who was told by the therapist that he seemed loving and friendly on Mondays and Wednesdays but acted like a whining tyrant on Saturdays (when he was brought by his parents instead of his housekeeper): He grinned, saying, "You don't know what I am like on Tuesdays and Thursdays!" In such cases, working toward the continuity and integration of the self-representation is an ongoing task that takes place both through the containment offered by the sessions and through verbalization of the contradictory self-images.

Working with the lack of ego and superego integration requires thorough discussion of contradictory behaviors in the therapeutic interaction. Splitting should be dealt with when it occurs within the session, as well as by contrasting information received from outside to what is observed in the session itself.

Support for Superego (Conscience) Integration

Another focus is working on the superego directly. While one child with superego lacunae was playing Pick-up-Sticks, the therapist asked him to watch whether he moved the sticks to see if he could tell her whether he had moved the sticks before she said anything. She could evaluate the functioning of his conscience by the promptness of his reports; at the same time, the therapist challenged him to check whether her conscience was working better or worse than his. This game was a very concrete way of practicing superego functions.

Support for Peer Relationships

The borderline child's lack of empathy for others is reflected in poor peer relations. In the therapeutic context, it is important to articulate what is happening to the relationship at all points, as if the therapist were an actual playmate. Although there are certainly countertransference risks in doing this approach, it is extremely useful in enabling the child to begin to work on social skills. Activity groups may be beneficially added for this purpose.

Objective Perception of Parents and Enhancement of Self-Reflective Capacity

The negative effects of the not-infrequent incidents of overt maternal rejection must be clarified by the therapist to the child in an attempt to sort out reality, fantasy, and the implications for realistic perceptions of oneself and of mother.

These interventions are best accepted if the therapist introduces them in an empathic manner. Borderline children's perceptions of different aspects of the maternal relationship, such as the child's expectations of unpredictability or rejection, should also be explained. Frequently these patients need to assess their parents' reality, including the parents' limitations as separate from themselves. In that way, they can come to grips with the parental environment without feeling that they are the cause or the victims of it. In other words, they need to enhance their capacity to reflect on their circumstances. This approach is particularly crucial in work with children who come from chaotic home environments. Grief for family deficit should be dealt with in therapy.

Resolution of Pre-Oedipal Conflicts

The various vicissitudes of pathological symbiosis and the conflicts around differentiation, practicing, and rapprochement need to be dealt with as they unfold in the transference. These difficulties correspond to the so-called pre-oedipal conflicts around issues of trust and distrust, remaining the same or becoming different, shadowing or darting away, coercing or being coerced, autonomy or dependence, being a boy or being a girl or being an undifferentiated neuter. These conflicts, their attendant anxieties (e.g., annihilation fears), and the primitive defenses (e.g., projection, denial, and splitting) should be spelled out in the treatment in the same way that neurotic conflicts with neurotic defenses are dealt with in less severe psychopathology.

Attenuation of Catastrophic Anxiety

Any potentially disruptive experience needs to be anticipated and verbalized because these children lack signal anxiety and thus are easily overwhelmed by abandonment anxiety or annihilation anxiety. Anxiety in these children needs to be articulated in terms of their omnipotent and magical fantasy thinking. Moves, hospitalizations, and impending parental divorces should be discussed as early as possible.

Borderline children need help in understanding their own deficits; those with such developmental deficits as ADHD need to recognize the nature of their handicap, their thoughts about it, its implications for their functioning, and its effects on their self-esteem. By talking realistically about the child's deficit, the therapist enables the child to acknowledge it, to share the knowledge with a trusted person, and to grieve. The child can then elaborate and resolve the fantasy systems in connections with the deficit. These fantasies usually are concerned with the child's feeling guilty or defective, and have thus contributed to the child's low self-esteem. Such a child needs help to learn how to compensate for the deficit by using his intact capacities.

Somatization

As borderline children are prone to various somatizations because of their dissociative tendencies and splitting, their use of body language needs to be clarified to them.

Impulsivity

Lack of impulse control seems to be a hallmark of borderline functioning, as is instability in the levels of ego organization. What is important, however, is that in children as in adults (O. Kernberg 1975), it may not necessarily represent an ego defect in the sense of lack of capacity to control, but it may be used defensively to manage anxiety. Clarification and interpretation of the purposes of poor impulse control may resolve what only may seem to be ego defects.

CLINICAL EXAMPLE

Norman, the elder of two siblings, came for consultation at the age of 7 after one year of treatment with a psychiatrist who saw him on a twice-weekly basis in addition to seeing his mother once a week. His previous psychotherapy had emphasized the verbalization of feelings to such an extent that he had been forbidden to play while in the treatment setting. He became worse, and by the time he came for consultation, he suffered from severe separation anxiety marked by an inability to sleep in his own room and an inability to be left alone day or night. In addition, Norman had no friends. Peer interaction was so bad that he was shunned by everybody in his elementary school. A school transfer was necessary because he was continually scapegoated and called names. Norman refused to bathe; he put his clothes on backwards and chewed his shirts. He presented occasional soiling and swallowed his nasal mucus as a matter of habit. He was depressed and moody. Although he was doing well academically in his new school, he fre-

174 BORDERLINE PERSONALITY DISORDER

quently talked about suicide—trying to get himself run over by a car, getting himself asphyxiated, taking pills, or falling off a building—all to the great distress of his parents.

There was severe marital tension between his parents, a professional couple. At the time of the consultation, they were talking about divorce, although they kept this information from the child.

Norman had been a planned child and an unusually "lovely baby." At the age of 2 years, 2 months, however, he had been seen by a specialist for developmental evaluation because he showed accelerated development in certain areas and retardation in others. His verbal functions, including vocabulary, comprehension, and complexity of speech, were quite advanced (as measured by the Bailey Scales and Stanford-Binet). In some of these tests he scored as high as 3 years. His perceptual and visual motor coordination were also accelerated. On tasks involving fine motor coordination, as well as items requiring prolonged attention, patience, and willingness to engage in activities not of his own choosing, his performance was more at the normal level. In contrast, his gross motor-control coordination was not well developed. He encountered difficulty in adapting his movements to different spatial configurations. For example, when his foot got caught beneath a chair, despite earnest efforts, he did not know how to free it. Nor did he know how to put his arms into the proper sleeves of his coat.

Although his intellectual abilities placed him in the superior range, he differed from the majority of 2-year-olds in the way he used them. His special interest in letters, shapes, writing, and reading was unusual, but from a developmental point of view, it was as much a liability as an asset. For one thing, his central nervous system had not matured to the point at which integrated and adaptive use of reading, writing, and even phonetic spelling could take place. He wrote with his left hand, reversed letters, and proceeded from right to left as well as vertically and randomly on the page. There was no clear-cut dominance with respect to a right/left preference of feet or eyes. In addition, certain features of Norman's behavior directly reflected tension and pressure. His writing and reciting of letters, for instance, became increasingly intense and erratic as his excitement mounted; the very fact that he turned to these activities when he was displeased or mildly frustrated for any reason indicated more than optimal tension.

Much could be said about Norman's disproportionate interest in shapes. It was as though he selectively perceived the form of the word at the expense of its functional meaning. In other words, he abstracted and conceptualized his environment to such a degree that his response to things did not match the perceptions and interests of other children. For him, blocks were primarily columns, triangles, and the like, or a means of constructing letters. Whereas for other children, blocks do have these properties, they are primarily potential houses, tunnels, or whatever. Nor was Norman able to use board games or rhythmic movement for imaginative play, although he could use them if these activities were supported by another person.

In summary, Norman showed precocity and age-appropriate development in certain areas. Yet lags in physical, social, and emotional development created an imbalance and made ego adaptation more difficult. He responded strongly to certain kinds of sensory and cognitive stimulation, but the extent to which his responses illustrated special vulnerability could not be assessed at the time. Already at 2 years, 2 months, he was considered to be at risk.

After his lack of response to the earlier treatments, Norman's therapy was started on an intensive psychoanalytic psychotherapy three times a week. Because this was a typical case of alternating parental neglect and indulgence, the parents received counseling every two or three weeks; in that forum, their belief that their secretiveness would protect the children from their marital tension was also addressed. (Part of Norman's insomnia stemmed from his overconcerns and conflicts about trying to keep his parents together. His father would watch him until he fell asleep.)

Norman began therapy in a rather apprehensive mood. During the first session, expecting to be subject to the rules from his previous therapy, he expressed his regret about not being allowed to play during the sessions. His new therapist explained that it didn't matter whether they talked or played; she wanted to get to know him so that she could help him understand his worries. He proceeded in the first few sessions to build a city with blocks. The first version contained a very narrow house that one could hardly get into and a saloon next door with a man watching through the window and a police truck in it. The second version included a wider, much more comfortable house in which two people could live and a helicopter entering a garage. The man in the saloon continued to watch through the window, but sometimes he came to the house to "relax." These, indeed, were the first indications of a therapeutic alliance with the therapist.

One session was of particular interest. Several times, Norman and the therapist had played Monopoly, which she interpreted as his way of controlling the number of things they could say or do. As he was setting up the pieces, he spontaneously remarked that he had tried to go to sleep between 8:30 and 9:30 P.M. the night before but that he had had to wait for three hours before his father came to his room to put him to bed. (Having his own bedroom was a new development, initiated at the therapist's suggestion.) She mentioned to Norman that she felt that he needed to see that he could fall asleep. He did not need to have his father there all night; his father could go once he fell asleep. "What happens when he doesn't come?" she asked. Norman mentioned seeing ghosts in the room. The therapist wondered what they looked like. According to Norman, they had see-saw mouths and dark eyes, were all black, and could stretch like chewing gum. When she asked him whether they were men or women, he answered that they were women ghosts. This response made the therapist wonder where his mother was in all this. He said that his mother was playing with the housekeeper, working on crossword puzzles. Norman paused and then added, "It makes me feel sad that she would prefer the puzzle better than me." The therapist then interpreted that he was probably afraid to be angry at her because she might really leave him; instead, he made up these ghosts to carry the anger, but he forgot that the ghosts were pretend and started thinking that the ghosts were angry at him, which of course frightened him. The therapist then said that he was hoping his mother would come, sticking to this wish year after year, not giving up. He wanted his mother to be available to him when he needed her, and it was hard and painful to see when she failed to do that; what was so hard to accept was that she didn't come of her own wishes. He said then that he was finished with his mother and wanted to play Monopoly.

At the end of the session, Norman went through the back door and for the first time asked the therapist just to count until he whistled, indicating that his housekeeper was there to accompany him. The therapist complied, telling him that if he didn't find the housekeeper, he could come back. He ventured into the relatively dark part of the patio, hopping along without fear, and did not need to return.

During this session, the therapist provided continuity through playing Monopoly. Norman had displaced his wish for someone to put him to sleep onto the father instead of the mother. (In fact, he had said that should his parents divorce, he would prefer to go with his father.) The therapist then observed that he had a hallucinatory experience with his ghosts. Knowing that he had the capacity to test reality, she insisted on his elaborating on this experience and sharing his thoughts with her. When she reacted to his fantasy with interest and without anxiety, his primary-process thinking could be replaced by secondary-process thinking. Specifically, he indicated what he was defending himself against when she asked him where his mother was in all this—namely, his depressed feeling about being second in importance to his mother's doing puzzles. After the therapist interpreted what he did with his ghosts, she became the target of the transference, namely, the mother of the rapprochement crisis. He was then able to ask the therapist, not his father or anybody else, to accompany him—symbolically—fulfilling his wish, without coercion, that she be available to him. He refueled by looking back briefly on his way out, but he could go through the dark part of the patio without her help, hopping along with an increased sense of autonomy and with less anxiety.

Norman's mother acknowledged that she had never had a moment of peace with him since the birth of his sibling when Norman was 2 years old. Norman had become so controlling, demanding, clinging, and negativistic that on many occasions she had told him she would send him away or that she would leave home as she actually did so from time to time.

Joint sessions with him and his mother were later instituted to deal with the stalemate in their relationship and his grief over it. One year later he ended the treatment with a significant improvement that enabled him to proceed with his development, as evidenced in a follow-up three years later.

SUMMARY

Therapeutic intervention requires a careful assessment of organic and psychological determinants in order to institute an appropriate treatment plan. This assessment is particularly important in children with borderline personality organization because of the frequent incidence of comorbidity with ADHD and depression.

The type of psychoanalytic psychotherapy recommended for borderline personality disorder focuses on clarification, confrontation, and interpretation of the here-and-now in the areas of transference, external reality, and the communicative process between therapist and patient. This process includes making the child cognizant of her organic deficits, if any, and enhancing her self-reflectiveness.

The interpretation of primitive defense mechanisms includes articulating their functions and the purposes of their use. The particular role of the therapist in facilitating the resolution of conflicts deriving from the separation/individuation stage is pivotal in this psychotherapeutic approach.

CONCLUSION

Most researchers believe that there is a continuity of borderline conditions into adulthood (Weil 1953). F. Pine (1974) described chronic failures in reality testing and object relations that prevail silently at all times in these children and go on to make for "the odd adult." Weil (1953) describes the same progression. Blum described such a continuity convincingly in his paper, "The Borderline Childhood of the Wolf Man" (1974). M. S. Mahler (1971), O. Kernberg (1975), and C. J. Kestenbaum (1983) also support this thesis. It is indeed justified if we assume that the borderline personality organization will remain insulated unless there is a therapeutic intervention intense and prolonged enough to change the internal world of the patient and enable him to modify his inner objects in accordance with external reality.

Borderline PD in children and adolescents is likely to have a common etiology. Differences between them stem more from the differences in developmental levels than from any differences in the intrinsic psychopathology of the borderline condition.

IV.3

Narcissistic Personality Disorder

DEFINITION

DSM-IV defines narcissistic personality disorder as "a pervasive pattern of grandiosity (in fantasy or behavior), need for admiration, and lack of empathy, beginning by early adulthood and present in a variety of contexts" (p. 661). Diagnosis in the adult patient requires evidence of at least five of the following:

grandiose sense of self-importance (whereby patient exaggerates achievements and talents and expects to be recognized as superior without commensurate achievements);

preoccupation with fantasies of unlimited success, power, brilliance, beauty, or ideal love;

belief that she is "special" and unique and can only be understood by, or should associate with, other special or high-status people (or institutions);

need for excessive admiration;

sense of entitlement (i.e., unreasonable expectations of especially favorable treatment or automatic compliance with own expectations);

interpersonal exploitation (for achievement of own ends);

lack of empathy; unwillingness to recognize or identify with the feelings and needs of others;

envy of others or conviction that others are envious of him; and

arrogant, haughty behaviors or attitudes.

DESCRIPTION

Although grandiose self-importance is central to narcissistic PD, vulnerability in self-esteem is an associated feature (*DSM-IV*). That hypersensibility makes narcissistic PD patients extremely sensitive to criticisms or failure, to which they may respond with disdain, rage, or defiant counterattack. Their endemic sense of entitlement is often reflected in impaired superego functioning, which presents as a lack of concern, guilt, or regret about the mistreatment of others. The resulting lapses in self-monitoring appear as antisocial traits; personal failings, defeats, or irresponsible behavior may be justified by rationalization, prevarication, or outright lying. Moreover, the primitive, persecutory destructive introjects that contribute to the formation of conscience but that have not been well-integrated into the narcissistic PD superego surface as paranoid anxieties projecting outwardly onto others or expressed inwardly as somatic and hypochondriacal symptoms. Finally, the unrelenting envy characteristic of the narcissistic PD patient destroys both the capacity to depend on others and the capacity to experience fulfillment with respect to one's own achievements or gratitude for what others have done.

The chronic intense envy and devaluation, the primitive idealization of self and others, the efforts toward omnipotent control, and the narcissistic withdrawal or aloofness are all defenses aimed at protecting the grandiose self. V. Volkvan (1973, 1979) has described in detail a number of defensive maneuvers used to protect the grandiose self from the assault of reality—the typical externalization of the conflict and restructuring of reality (i.e., blaming others), the glass-bubble fantasy (surrounding oneself with a wall of aloofness), and the use of transitional fantasies (e.g., day dreams of self-aggrandizement).

COMPARATIVE PERSPECTIVES

NORMAL NARCISSISM AND NARCISSISTIC PERSONALITY DISORDER

It is important to contrast the pathological self-centeredness of narcissistic PD children with what is considered the normal narcissism of childhood. In normal narcissism, the child's need for dependence and admiration is fulfilled by the age-appropriate attention he receives; he is able to acknowledge nurturing with reciprocity and gratitude. The child with a narcissistic pathology denies her dependence, however; she receives nurturance with a sense of entitlement and does not reciprocate or experience any sense of gratitude.

In normal infantile narcissism, the tendency to claim exaggerated achievements and talents involves playful fantasies of being a superachiever or having extraordinary powers: The child plays at being Superman. In the pathological case of narcissistic PD, the child strongly believes he has already achieved what he wishes to be; there is nothing playful in this experience (viz., the child called Matt who matter-of-factly refers to himself as "SuperMatt," Egan and Kernberg 1984).

The child's grandiose sense of self is the fusion of the positive aspects of the actual self, the ideal self, and ideal role models; anything incompatible is eliminated (Figure IVf), so what is left is a highly exaggerated self-image. There is no room for anyone else to be special too. On the contrary, everybody else has to be inferior; the child needs to control or to destroy his own achievement (e.g., the boy who tore up his own award certificate on learning that his schoolmate got one too). In contrast to the normal infantile competitiveness of the child who learns to tolerate losing in order to preserve her relationship with parent or friend, the narcissistic PD child competes to eliminate her rival.

The normal child's dependency and demands on the environment correspond to realistic expectations and can be fulfilled. The narcissistic PD child's demands are excessive and therefore coercive, precluding any sense of gratification and appreciation and triggering anger in the caretaker who feels imposed upon to meet them. Supplies are never sufficient to satisfy the demands of the grandiose self, so no matter how much is given, the child still feels unloved. In addition, he experiences envy because he is not the sole center of all that is good; there are others who have things he wants. This envy impairs his capacity to receive even nurturance and experience fulfillment without resentment.

Whereas normal children show genuine attachments to, and interest in, others and can trust and depend on the significant adults in their lives, those with pathological narcissism can neither trust nor depend beyond the immediate context of need-gratification. Even a normal 2-year-old can maintain a positive investment in mother during brief separations, but the child with narcissistic PD has only unstable attachments, subject to change with the advent of a minor frustration.

Narcissistic personalities are especially vulnerable to frustration or criticism because of their need to be the best. Moreover, the burden of sustaining specialness exposes them to extra confrontations with painful everyday frustrations. They require excessive and constant admiration to feel good about themselves because they suffer from a pathological form of self-esteem regulation, whereas normal narcissism with normal self-esteem regulation leads to realistic self-acceptance (i.e., of negative as well as positive qualities).

The normal person derives gratification from actual accomplishments and also from investing effort toward reaching her goals. Because a healthy tension prevails among the actual self, the ideal self, and ideal role models, the individual's conscience permits her to feel rewarded when she achieves. She can, of course, recognize others' achievements as well. The narcissistic PD patient, who is already his own ideal, goes through a very different experience: He has to disown everything that does not fit with his grandiose sense of self, which means he must perceive others in a distorted way. They are devalued and feared due to the lack of integration of the self caused by splitting (Figure IVf).

ASSOCIATION WITH OTHER DSM-IV DISORDERS, AXIS I AND AXIS II

Comorbidity with depression and dysthymia, substance abuse, and bipolar disorder appears in adults (Ronningstam 1998). In children and adolescents, narcissistic PD coexists clinically with depressive disorders, anxiety disorders (especially separation anxiety), oppositional defiant disorders, and phobias. (In hospitalized youngsters, who exhibit the most severe forms of pathological narcissism, anorexia nervosa and disruptive disorders occur with particular frequency.)

There is a 50 percent overlap between narcissistic and borderline PDs in adults. According to one study (Morey 1988), adults with narcissistic PD are five times more likely to have antisocial PDs as well; where there is overlap with antisocial behavior, the prognosis is markedly worse. In children, there are clinical reports of overlap with borderline and antisocial PDs.

DEVELOPMENTAL PSYCHOPATHOLOGY

The adult criteria for narcissistic PD outlined in DSM-IV have direct parallels in the childhood incarnation, as evidenced by Matt, who denoted his

Normal Narcissism

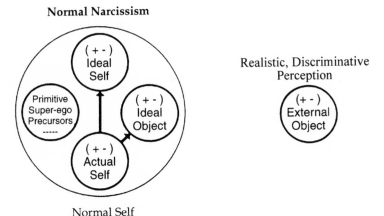

Realistic, Discriminative
Perception

Normal Self

FIGURE IVf1   Normal self-esteem regulation

Pathological Narcissism

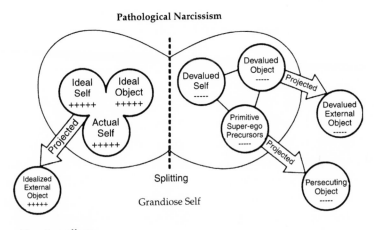

Grandiose Self

- : Negative affects
+ : Positive affects
(+ -) : There is no integration of positive and negative affects

FIGURE IVf2   Pathological self-esteem regulation

sense of unlimited power by calling himself SuperMatt. He expected to be recognized as superior when he, The Boss, called his employees to come to his house. That he expected them to report instantly illustrated his sense of entitlement, his lack of empathy, and his devaluation of them. When he posed "algebra equations" on the blackboard, he demonstrated haughty arrogance by summarily rejecting all answers as stupid. In the course of asserting omnipotent control, Matt sought to devalue his therapist—who could barely stand his fault-finding and other derogatory remarks. All of these characteristics are reflected in the child's self-esteem; in his patterns of interaction with family, friends, and peers; and in his school performance.

Self-esteem. It is the paradox between his self-centeredness or heightened sense of himself, which manifests as arrogance, and his extreme vulnerability and hypersensitivity to criticism that puts his self-esteem into a chronically precarious equilibrium. He cannot tolerate the frustration of having to accommodate to environmental constraints that threaten his grandiosity.

Interactions. Because of his exaggerated sense of self-importance, the narcissistic PD child is unable to appreciate or to empathize with others; because of his sense of entitlement, he is exploitative and also has a low frustration threshold. These traits lead to a propensity for manipulativeness, lying, stealing, and other antisocial behaviors, which lead in turn to rejection by his peers. His envy of others' fun and his reactive aloofness, as well as his intolerance of differences between himself and others, result in rejection as well. The reciprocity normally expected during school-age years is practically nonexistent; in consequence, peer relationships are seriously impaired.

Academic performance. Children with narcissistic PD do not enjoy their learning experiences. They are frequently good students, but their achievements are aimed at eliciting admiration from others rather than at acquiring knowledge for its intrinsic value or personal benefit. As admiration for their performance wanes, so does their interest in the subject; boredom prevails.

Pathologically narcissistic children's pattern of fluctuating performance can also be explained by the sense of entitlement: They do not find it easy to apply themselves to mastering a new subject and get poor grades due to lack of effort. They develop a functional learning disability that has a profile quite different from the classic kind, which derives from neuropsychological deficits.

Gaze aversion. The inability or refusal to have eye contact may have multiple determinants. It seems to be serving the illusion of specialness: By literally not looking around, the patient avoids comparing himself with others. It may stem as well from early discordance between the child and the caregiver's perception of the child, whereby she does not receive full emotional acknowledgment of her separateness and individuality. By averting her gaze, the child avoids the pain of not being recognized. Gaze aversion also facilitates avoidance of critical judgments and other unwelcome expectations.

Selective deafness or tuning out. As a way to preserve the integrity of the grandiose self, children with narcissistic pathology may selectively tune out an invasive parent. The invasiveness may lie not only in the content of the parent's words but also in the unrelentingness of verbal barrage: The sound, the rhythm, the timing, and the substantive appropriateness all determine the child's receptiveness to verbal interventions. Not surprisingly, the child may extend the pattern to "turning off" his therapist. Both parent and therapist may, in turn, often respond by withdrawing—which increases the child's sense of abandonment and deprivation and catalyzes his narcissistic defenses. The ensuing vicious cycle chronically sequesters the narcissistic child, who—instead of being contained in a sound envelope that can hold him emotionally like a mother's gaze—becomes selectively "deaf" to others as he has become selectively "blind."

Play pathology. Narcissistic children show a marked inhibition of play, which is expressed initially as boredom; indeed, they will quickly complain that there are no worthwhile toys in the playroom during the assessment, for example. This phenomenon has psychodynamic roots. Devaluation protects her inflated sense of self: It is not she who has problems in play but the toys that are not good. The claim of boredom disguises the threat to the grandiose self represented by the possibility of defeat in structured games, and also avoids the attendant risk of rages or temper tantrums. Also, it fends off the primitive aggression fantasies that surface in treatment when the narcissistic child sadistically plays scenarios where she dismantles, dismembers, and massacres doll figures.

Separation anxiety. The high level of separation anxiety in narcissistic youngsters presents another paradox. The same child who shows himself as entitled, important, and powerful is extremely vulnerable to being alone: He cannot let go of his caregiver, finds it difficult to leave the house, cannot go away to camp, or cannot even participate in sleep-overs.

Because the caregiver's presence serves as an auxiliary support that the child takes for granted as an extension of his grandiose self, parents are also frequently apprehensive as to how their child will function without them. The separation anxiety is not often addressed as a chief complaint, however, because the child's grandiosity diverts the clinician's attention to aspects other than the sense of frailty the child experiences when confronted with separation or being alone.

Preoccupation with self-image. The youngster with narcissistic PD is frequently obsessed with her reflection in the mirror. In some cases, a mirror addiction develops, whereby the child spends a long time looking at herself in a compulsive manner as if the mirror could give her feedback as to who and what she is. The fact that the need to look in the mirror is never satisfied reflects a lack of positive and reciprocal gaze-interaction with the human mirror, the caregiver (P. Kernberg 1987).

Justin's Reflection, E. Broussard's 1983 videotape following a boy from 18 months to 4 years of age shows that Justin has no eye contact with his mother. He shows such fascination with his mirror image that he spends long periods of time looking at himself and his gestures while excluding others, including the examiner. Indeed, Justin's mother rarely acknowledged his needs, wants, or distress; she seemed to recognize her son only when they were engaged in a mutually seductive interaction. Justin built up a grandiose self to protect himself from his psychological pain, and in a follow-up assessment at the age of 17, he presented a full-fledged narcissistic PD.

ADOLESCENT NARCISSISTIC PERSONALITY DISORDER

In a review of adolescent inpatient records, P. F. Kernberg and colleagues (1998) found moderate to high levels of narcissism even in the almost 50 percent of cases whose discharge diagnosis showed no personality disorder, using a modified version of J. Gunderson and colleagues' (1990) diagnostic criteria. The severity was greater, of course, among the patients ultimately identified as having narcissistic PDs. Distribution between boys and girls was equal, but boys tended to be more boastful and pretentious and to show more disregard for conventional rules and values, whereas girls tended even more significantly to react with detachment; pseudo-indifference; and aloofness in response to criticism, defeat, disappointment, or separation.

The sexuality of narcissistic PD adolescents revealed a high degree of exhibitionism. The subjects either did not date or dated for the purpose of showing off, choosing the most popular, attractive, perfect partners as trophies; at times, however, they associated with the least desirable instead so as to shine by comparison and also to enlist an unconditional and grateful admirer.

Overall, 90 percent of the variance in inpatient narcissistic PD diagnosis was cumulatively accounted for by the quality of the adolescent's interpersonal relations (53 percent); his grandiosity and reactiveness, as derived from a scale related to hypersensitivity (88 percent); and combined moral and social adaptation (91 percent).

PSYCHOLOGICAL TESTING AND DIAGNOSTIC ASSESSMENT

PSYCHOLOGICAL TESTING

Projective testing may validate an independent diagnosis of narcissistic PD. On the Child Apperception Test, for example, D. M. Abrams (1993) reported that heroes are ineffectual, wimpy, and overwhelmed; father figures are mostly immature, incompetent, boastful buffoons; mother figures range from nurturing to unprotective to critical, immature, and self-centered; peers are largely undifferentiated or acting in parallel or subservient fashion. Percepts of junior figures do not appear: Their omission is consistent with the pathologically narcissistic child's intense problems with sibling rivalry that can easily become outright abuse. All cognitive functions seem to be intact, but control of drives, mastery competence, and defensive operations are deficient and immature. Moreover, in terms of object relations, the test reveals little differentiation among people, who emerge as shadowy, vague, and exaggerated figures instead of distinct individual identities.

A study of 36 narcissistic PD children (ages 6–12) showed their tendency to be positive on several of the Exner constellations (Bardenstein 1998). They exhibit a capacity to distort reality and to engage in peculiar or thought-disordered ideation; further, they show diminished ability to see conventional reality. The findings also indicate that faulty or distorted reasoning further impairs the children's functioning. The Hypervigilance Index (HVI) suggests that narcissistic PD children invest significant energy in protecting the self against the perceived malevolence of the outside world; they are interpersonally guarded, remaining suspicious of others' motives, and they zealously maintain personal space. Although extremely rare in nonpatient children and adolescents, the HVI constellations distinguished the narcissistic PD population over 7 years of age. On the Coping Deficit Index (CDI), a measure of general copying capacity, a majority was positive as well, particularly in the interpersonal realm. A positive CDI is associated with interpersonal ineptness and a chaotic history of relationships. The Depression Index (DEPI) was also elevated, suggesting incidence of dysphoric affect, low self-esteem, and psychological pain not consistently evident in the patients' presenting symptoms.

A high number of space responses on the Rorschach Test correlates with an alienated, oppositional stance that can lead to clashes with others in the environment. Anger and resentment are triggered easily; the choice of the nonconformist role is additionally distancing. The cognitive process also appears to succumb to the need to protect the self, as narcissistic PD children turn to their own ideation as their best resource for solving problems or addressing demands. Their susceptibility to simplifying and distorting information, however, seriously compromises the efficiency of their problem-solving style. All of these constellations, again rare in nonpatient comparison groups, represent premature, crystallized developmental formations that are stable over time and unlikely to disappear with continued maturation (Erdberg 1996).

FAMILY CHARACTERISTICS AND DYNAMICS IN THE CASE OF A CHILD WITH NARCISSISTIC PERSONALITY DISORDER

Matt, the boy introduced earlier, was 8 years old when he came for a diagnostic evaluation. The elder of two brothers, he was friendless because he acted selfish, domineering, and entitled: He ordered other children about as though they were his slaves (and in fact called those who worked with him on a neighborhood paper his "employees").

Although he was intelligent and had no organic impairments, his achievements were significantly below his potential. He did not participate in any sports—he would not swim, skate, ride a bike, or throw a ball—and was unable to face up to the fact that learning these skills would require an effort on his part. Indeed, he was reluctant to exert any effort because he would feel deeply humiliated if he did not meet with immediate success. His boastfulness and sense of entitlement drove him to disavow any misbehavior by lying and by becoming aloof.

He physically tortured his brother, who had been born after a long hiatus deriving from the parents' concern about inflicting a sibling on their firstborn. His mother focused her attentions on Matt, attempting to fulfill her own hopes through him. She was the dominant figure in the family, and Matt identified with her style in attempting to dominate his peers. His mother's administrative and executive talents made her a prominent member of the community, but they translated into controlling Matt in all his waking hours—in what he ate (Halloween candy was to be enjoyed one piece per day, so that Matt was still eating it the next May) and on his bedtime, such that Matt was forced to go to sleep at 8 P.M. regardless of whether or not he was in the midst of doing something. He had to develop a grandiose self and other narcissistic defenses against the intrusion of, and utter control by, his mother.

In spite of his serious difficulties in daily life, particularly his lack of friendships, Matt denied any problem and repeatedly insulted and devalued his therapist. He aimed to make the therapist look stupid and said as much; he continually conveyed his sense of boredom and irritation at having to come to sessions. By age 8, he already fulfilled the criteria for narcissistic PD, including the stability of his traits across time and across situations.

Matt's family dynamics and family structure illustrate some of the characteristics of the parents of narcissistic PD children. Mother was herself a narcissistic person who idealized her child and did not acknowledge his vulnerabilities: She saw him only as an agent to gratify her own self-esteem. Father was passive and seemed to be a marginal authority.

The parents animated D. Rinsley's description (1989): They facilitated a sense of individuation in terms of achievements but did not facilitate a sense of separation. The child could not function as an autonomous person, nor could he even experience himself as such. In this connection, adopted children, abusive children, overindulged or wealthy children, and children of divorce may be at risk for the same psychopathology. In each of these special situations, the child may be considered an extension of parental wishes and needs, not free to separate and function autonomously. (If he is assigned the role of replacing the father, as is sometimes the case after divorce, the normal infantile desire to compete against the same-sex parent is corrupted. If instead the parent wants to eradicate all traits of the former marital partner in the child, the child may have to develop a sense of grandiosity and entitlement to protect himself from such interference with his own autonomous self.) In the case of the overindulged or physically handicapped child, normal infantile narcissism may be prolonged.

The narcissistic personality syndrome might also be precipitated by the dependent, insecure mother who wants her child to behave absolutely perfectly to increase her own self-esteem; the father who seems to be unable to establish his authority and appears extremely indulgent and unable to set consistent limits; parental intrusiveness and overinvolvement that disallow the child's development of a sense of his own body and his separate self; parents who cannot assert generational boundaries and consequently neglect the child's need to outgrow his infantile omnipotence; parents who do not provide feedback and do not convey their emotional availability to the child, forcing him to become his own (ideal) parent in compensation; parents who are reluctant to criticize a child's behavior at the risk of hurting his feelings, thereby failing to give him clear standards and to establish a superego; and parents who do not confront the child when he behaves disrespectfully, as if kid gloves would appease the child/monster (viz., the mother who meekly apologizes for running out of orange juice when an enraged child demands it, but never addresses the aggressive demeanor of the child, who internalizes himself as a terror whom no one can dare to control).

TREATMENT

The aim of treatment is the transformation of the patient's pathological narcissism into a normal infantile narcissism in the case of a child, or normal narcissism in the case of an adolescent. Essentially, the various maladaptive forms of self-esteem regulation should be addressed in such a way that sources of gratification and self-reward promote rather than interfere with emotional development. The therapist must have both a psychodynamic background as well as a developmental understanding of the factors entering into the pathology so that interventions can be focused at the development level of the patient as well as on the particular personality pathology.

Individual therapy. Insight-oriented psychoanalytic treatment is recommended with a minimum of two to four weekly sessions.

One important objective is to resolve the grandiosity of self-centeredness. The personality structure that H. Kohut (1971, 1972) described as the grandiose self accounts for most of the criteria outlined by *DSM-IV*—the grandiose sense of self-importance, preoccupation with fantasies of unlimited success, feelings of uniqueness and entitlement, exploitativeness, arrogance and haughtiness. These traits unfold in the course of the relationship with the therapist, and when they are identified, the patient can confront her maladaptive solutions while acquiring alternative approaches to meet her needs for positive self-esteem and self-regard. The patient should be helped to see the limitations of her own approaches and to begin to distinguish her real self from her idealized version and accept it. The patient should also be helped to discover how to replace her grandiose hopes with realistically achievable ones. She should also be helped to recognize, without suffering destructive and alienating envy, that others have qualities of value.

The next objective is to exchange the immature defense mechanisms that maintain this pathology for higher-level coping mechanisms. Narcissistic PD patients resort to splitting, denial, idealization, omnipotent control, projective identification, and (most characteristic) devaluation (O. Kernberg 1975) in order to protect their grandiosity. These defenses weaken the ego's capacities and therefore the patient's effective adaptation to others and to his surroundings; because they are expressed interpersonally, they also result in impaired interactions. The other is induced, through role responsiveness (Sandler 1976), to act as a controlling, devalued victim; the outcome is conflict and rupture. Work with these personality traits requires tact and empathy because of the vulnerability of the patient's self-esteem; patients may drop out of treatment or become intensely depressed or act out if confronted without care-appropriate sense of timing.

A third objective is to identify and to address the patient's need to understand her characterological depression in terms of her progressive realization that her illusions of self-sufficiency, achievement, and relationships have been illusions, indeed, the products of her grandiosity. The patient will have to face and explore her self-deception and maladaptation.

The fourth objective is to work on age-appropriate peer relationships. The capacity to maintain friendships is pivotal to self-esteem regulation. The therapist must bring out the patient's tolerance and empathy so he can handle not being the exclusive center of attention and can recognize and execute reciprocal exchanges.

Resolving separation anxiety is yet another objective. Working on the grandiosity, primitive defense mechanisms, and peer relations may increase autonomy and improve adaptation. Targeted medications during this transition period may be helpful.

Narcissistic transferences. The therapist must work tactfully to make the child realize the disadvantages of sustaining her grandiosity. To this end, the therapist may point out paradigms unfolding in the therapeutic relationship—for example, the patient's tendency to feel that she is a twin of the therapist, the ways in which she eliminates differences from the therapist that make her feel envious, the need either to elicit the unconditional admiration of the therapist to magnify her own self-esteem or to regard the therapist as admirable and all-powerful in order to bask in the therapist's reflected glory, the need to devalue the therapist, and the conviction that she can be her own better therapist. H. Kohut (1971, 1972) described all of these paradigms as narcissistic transferences; they operate in children as well as in adults. When worked through with the child so that he can see them as distorted and illusory forms of relating with real disadvantages, the child can gradually give up his immature interactions, defenses, or coping styles and can resume his healthy development.

Countertransference. The effectiveness of therapy may be threatened by the fact that narcissistic PD patients tend to provoke rejection and withdrawal in the therapist in the face of devaluation, aggression, and envy. Moreover, the therapist may submit to the patient's grandiosity and omnipotent control by trying to appease the patient rather than by attacking the problematic interactions directly. The therapist is at constant risk of falling into the aforementioned complementary role responsiveness (Sandler 1976) evoked by the child or adolescent's verbal and nonverbal behavior.

Group therapy. Work with the interpersonal dynamics that emerge not only between the group therapist and the patient but among peers in the small group may be quite effective for youngsters whose social skills are severely impaired. Psychodynamic in its theoretical framework, this intervention also addresses developmental appropriateness in friendship and peer interactions.

Family therapy. To the extent that family interactions sustain the patient's pathology—for example, by appeasing and submitting to, or contrarily by withdrawing from, defensive devaluation, idealization, and omnipotence—family therapy can be a useful modality. The same psychodynamic theory that informs individual therapy is applied to family therapy techniques (Berkowitz et al. 1974). Family therapy may be a productive adjunct if the patient can only be seen once a week individually. In this forum, parents can learn to set limits to the child's grandiosity and avoid fueling his personality pathology.

CONCLUSION

The prognosis for childhood narcissistic PD has improved significantly, thanks to better psychodynamic understanding of its etiology and to the development of specific psychotherapeutic strategies.

IV.4

Antisocial Personality Disorder

In 1993 two boys, both 11, abducted a two-year-old from a shopping center in the outskirts of Liverpool, England. They tried to push him into a nearby canal, then dragged him two-and-a-half miles to a railway embankment. They threw stones and bricks at him, kicked him in the head, and bludgeoned him with a 22-pound iron bar. They then tried to disguise their acts as an accident by laying the child's dead body on the rail, where it was cut in two by a passing train. One of the children, according to the journalist's report, "showed a disturbing lack of remorse." Both boys were "truants from broken homes in a rough neighborhood."

—Newsweek, December 6, 1993, p. 15

DEFINITION

In the United States, juvenile murders are the cause of death of 10 people a day. The average age of these mostly male murderers, who kill with weapons (usually firearms), is 14.7 years. The category of antisocial personality disorder (ASPD) is not recognized in *DSM-IV* for anyone under age 18, however. Children and adolescents who display ASPD characteristics are most commonly diagnosed with conduct disorder.

Indeed, having had a conduct disorder before the age of 15 is one of the essential criteria for the eventual diagnosis of antisocial PD. One study has identified those patients with ASPD as those who have been antisocial since early childhood (Moffitt 1993). As indicated by the following *DSM-IV* tables,

193

the criteria for antisocial PD in adults correspond to the criteria for conduct disorder in children.

Figures IVg (1) and (2) reproduce the descriptions in *DSM-IV* of the characteristics of adult ASPD and conduct disorders in children, respectively. All seven adult criteria are represented in the child conduct disorder.

Adult failure to conform to social norms with respect to unlawful behaviors corresponds in the child to lying, threatening, and intimidation (1); stealing while confronting a victim (mugging, purse snatching, extortion, armed robbery) (6); and forcing someone into sexual activity (7).

Deceitfulness as indicated by repeated lying, use of aliases, or conning others for personal profit or pleasure is paralleled by frequent lying or conning others to obtain goods or favors or to avoid obligations (11).

Impulsivity and/or failure to plan ahead is echoed in the diagnostic table for conduct disorders by staying out at night contrary to parental prohibitions as early as age 13 (13), by having run away from home at least twice overnight or at least once for a longer period (14), and by frequent truancy beginning before age 14 (15).

FIGURE IVg(1)   Antisocial Personality Disorder

Cluster B Personality Disorders
•301.7 Antisocial Personality Disorder
A. There is a pervasive pattern of disregard for and violation of the rights of others occurring since age 15 years, as indicated by three or more of the following:

    (1) failure to conform to social norms with respect to lawful behaviors as indicated by repeatedly performing acts that are grounds for arrest
    (2) deceitfulness as indicated by repeated lying, use of aliases, or conning others for personal profit or pleasure
    (3) impulsivity or failure to plan ahead
    (4) irritability and aggressiveness, as indicated by repeated physical fights or assault
    (5) reckless disregard for safety of self or others
    (6) consistent irresponsibility, as indicated by repeated failure to sustain consistent work behavior or honor financial obligations
    (7) lack of remorse, as indicated by being indifferent to or rationalizing having hurt, mistreated, or stolen from another

B. The individual is at least age 18 years.
C. There is evidence of Conduct Disorder (see p. 66) with onset before age 15 years.
D. The occurence of antisocial behavior is not exclusively during the course of Schizophrenia or a Manic Episode.

FIGURE IVg(2)   Conduct Disorder

•312.8 Conduct Disorder
A.   A repetitive and persistent pattern of behavior in which the basic rights of others or major age-appropriate societal norms or rules are violated, as manifested by the presence of three (or more) of the following criteria in the past 12 months, with at least one criterion present in the past 6 months.

   (1)   often bullies, threatens, or intimidates others
   (2)   often initiates physical fights
   (3)   has used a weapon that can cause serious physical harm to others (e.g., a bat, brick, broken bottle, knife, gun)
   (4)   has been physically cruel to people
   (5)   has been physically cruel to animals
   (6)   has stolen while confronting a victim (e.g., mugging, purse snatching, extortion, armed robbery)
   (7)   has forced someone into sexual activity
   (8)   has deliberately engaged in fire setting with the intention of causing serious damage
   (9)   has deliberately destroyed others' property (other than by fire setting)
  (10)   had broken into someone else's house, building, or car
  (11)   often lies to obtain goods or favors or to avoid obligations (i.e., "cons" others)
  (12)   has stolen items of nontrivial value without confronting a victim (e.g., shoplifting, but without breaking and entering; forgery)
  (13)   often stays out at night despite parental prohibitions, beginning before age 13 years
  (14)   has run away from home overnight at least twice while living in parental or parental surrogate home (or once without returning for a lengthy period)
  (15)   often truant from school, beginning before age 14
  (16)   from DSMIV-CD Model case: 15 year old Joe "accused by a female classmate of forcing her to have sex with him. He replied that she agreed to have sex with him and then got angry with him because he went out with other girls."

B.   The disturbance in behavior causes clinically significant impairment in social, academic, or occupational functioning.
C.   If the individual is age 18 years or older, criteria are not met for Antisocial Personality Disorder.

Specify type based on age at onset:
Childhood-Onset Type: onset of at least one criterion characteristic of Conduct Disorder prior to age 10 years.
Adolescent-Onset Type: absence of any criteria characteristic of Conduct Disorder prior to age 10 years.

(continues)

FIGURE IVg(2) *(continued)*

Specify severity:

Mild: few if any conduct problems in excess of those required to make the diagnosis and conduct problems cause only minor harm to other (e.g., lying, truancy, staying out after dark without permission.

Moderate: number of conduct problems and effect on other intermediate between "mild" and "severe" (e.g., stealing without confronting a victim; vandalism)

Severe: many conduct problems in excess of those required to make the diagnosis or conduct problems cause considerable harm to others (e.g., forced sex, physical cruelty, use of a weapon, stealing while confronting a victim; breaking and entering)

Irritability and aggressiveness in adult ASPD as signaled by repeated physical fights or assaults compares to the child or adolescent's propensities to initiate physical fights (3) and use a weapon that can cause serious physical harm (3).

Reckless disregard for safety of self or others matches physical cruelty in children to people (4) and animals (5).

Consistent irresponsibility (e.g., repeated failure to honor work or financial obligations) is reflected in truancy (15) once again.

Lack of remorse, as represented by indifference to or rationalizing having hurt, mistreated, or stolen from another, resonates with the *DSM-IV* model case for conduct disorder in which a 15-year-old boy accused of rape contended that the victim resented his going out with other girls and anyway had agreed to have sex with him (16).

DESCRIPTION

Three cases of different developmental levels and different severity will illustrate the traits characteristic of antisocial personality disorder—excepting, of course, the criterion of age.

A 6-YEAR-OLD BOY

Herman was the elder of two siblings; his brother was 4 years old. Herman was brought in for evaluation because he was bullying other children, destroying their property, stealing money and other possessions from peers as well as from family, and lying at school and at home. He flouted authority and was impervious to discipline or rewards. Herman physically tortured his brother, bending his arms and attempting to throw him down the stairs; he also abused his brother verbally, telling him that he wished he were dead, that he did not belong to the family, and that he would cut him into pieces. On one occasion, when Herman was introduced to a neighborhood boy for the first time, he stepped on a pet guinea pig that the boy was holding in his hands.

Herman came from an intact family. His mother's pregnancy and delivery were uneventful; he was breast-fed and met the regular developmental landmarks. He was described as having been extremely active and aggressive as long as the parents could remember so that from the time he walked, he became a challenge to their limit-setting. The father commented that his son had "a most criminal mind" and that if he grew up the way he was at that moment "he would become a real danger"—even that "without treatment he would turn into an assassin." The mother, a patient and caring woman in her middle thirties, felt exhausted by the demands of her older son, who could not be left alone for fear he would torture his brother or destroy property in the house. Herman would alternately cling to his mother, kissing her in a demanding, manipulative way, and call her stupid and dumb when she did not meet his demands.

On rare occasions Herman was able to talk about his feelings and his subjective experience. Thus, he said once that he would like to "choke his brother, cut his head off with the sharpest knife, and give him to his parents to eat." He talked of his hatred of girls and how he and a friend with similar personality characteristics would put spikes from tree branches on the sand so that the girls at school who passed by would fall and hurt themselves. He noted that "in a bad world he would choke girls off and turn them into mashed potatoes or he could cut all girls into pieces and send them into outer space. . . . In a bad world you either get killed or kill." He added that sometimes a feeling came, "I can't explain it," a feeling of "being sad, there is nothing to do, it is a blank world with no Adam, no Eve, no grass, like made of wax."

This child did not show psychotic behaviors, nor did he suffer from delusions or hallucinations. His statement revealed his aloneness and the paranoid experience of being in a world where everybody was out for the kill. His extreme isolation and the frozen nature of this barren world illustrate the almost total absence of an affective investment in other people.

Herman's comments about the contrast between the rules of a good world and those of a bad world were made in the presence of his mother: They signaled his awareness of what she might want to hear and his attempt to comply with her expectations, parroting rather than internalizing the values as his own.

He perceived the usual playground activity of girls chasing boys in a paranoid framework: "The girls want to chase us and kill us, to pay us back for what we did to them." A child like Herman turns developmentally appropriate play between boys and girls into an aggressive event with no playful quality at all.

A thin line separated Herman from the child murderers in Jonesboro, Arkansas, who in 1998 at the ages of 10 and 11 made careful plans to massacre schoolmates with a machine gun. They placed themselves in a strategic position where the children had to pass by as they left the building after the boys set off the fire alarm. All of this was done with premeditation. Herman was acting on just such murderous impulses at the age of 6 when he tortured his younger sibling physically and psychologically. By age 8, he was constructing play scenes of interplanetary battles in which dinosaurs would declare humans disgusting, smelly, and stupid; the human figures were smothered to death under a coat of Play-Dough and all their cats and dogs were bombed. He would then proclaim, "Everybody is dead (under) the shower of death." With treatment, Herman became progressively able to play with the theme of death rather than carry his murderous impulses into action, and he was no longer expelled from schools and summer camps where he was now able to establish friendships.

A 10-YEAR-OLD GIRL

Maggie was an African American child with a stormy history. She was described as irritable, aggressive, threatening, and assaultive toward her 7-year-old brother, whom she had burned with a light bulb on the weekend prior to her admission. She came in with the chief complaint, "I am scared." Maggie also threatened and assaulted her peers and had outbursts of temper, a long record of lying and stealing, especially from her mother, and suicidal ideation; she had attempted to jump out of a second-story school window earlier that year. Medications, including Ritalin, Mellaril, Klonopin, Tegretol, Propranolol, and Valproate, had had no effect.

She was born when her mother was 13 years old. Her mother married at 19 after abandonment by a common-law husband; the new husband was killed in a drive-by shooting that Maggie witnessed.

During contacts with adults, she was characteristically uncooperative and aloof. She was manipulative, demanding and defiant, angry, and sullen, as well as provocative. Throughout her hospitalization, she continued to be threatening, aggressive, and unresponsive to directions and discipline.

After her discharge to a special residential setting, Maggie was seen to "bond better with the teacher, develop trust," and although she had difficult days, the school felt that they could work with her. This report by the primary therapist assigned to that school was written only two weeks after Maggie left the hospital, where she had been essentially unchanged since admission. It is unlikely that she would have achieved that amount of transformation, however; as is characteristic in these cases, the hope for change seems to be more a reflection of the good wishes of the mental health professional than the actual objective status of the patient. It is common for the adults surrounding such children to express good faith, attribute distress to them, and minimize the severity of their acts (Myers 1995). For example, "this child would be considered antisocial personality were it not that she is in the process of development Her behavior would have a bad prognosis, but occasionally she states she is sorry . . . ".

AN ADOLESCENT GIRL

Joanne was a 16-year-old female who had been adopted at one week of age. Her two younger siblings were the biological children of her middle-aged professional parents. During her elementary school years, she suffered from petit mal epilepsy and was classified as learning disabled, requiring special education programs. In the early grades, her school work was inconsistent; in high school, she did well in subjects she liked and failed the ones she disliked. She rejected history, for instance, because the study of "dead people" was of no use to her.

She displayed temper outbursts and cruelty to other children her age. She once broke another child's arm. The parents were afraid to leave her alone with her younger siblings. At 15 she became pregnant by a man in his early twenties, a known drug dealer, and had an abortion. She ran away from home several times, on one occasion living for several months "as a homeless person" with her boyfriend. She was arrested by police for breaking into and burglarizing a home. Her stealing began during elementary school, and she was described as having lied since she was a small child. She behaved impulsively and did not show remorse. She did not have close girlfriends; her only friends were male.

As an adolescent, Joanne was attractive, but she had a coarse, vulgar manner and appeared dejected and bitter. Her language was sparse, partly because of problems in understanding what was said to her and partly because she withheld information ("I'm not saying yes, and I'm not saying no"). She spoke in a low tone, her utterances garbled, and did not volunteer any information; she addressed a topic only when she realized that the interviewer had foreknowledge about it. She acted indifferent and cynical. Her attitude toward adults was colored by distrust. In her interactions with professionals and parents, she was dismissive and derogatory. When faced with situations where guilt or remorse would be the expected reaction, she would profess not to know the meaning of those feelings: "What's that?" Overall, there was a sense of hopelessness about her future. "I take it a day at a time; I go with the flow." In her relationship with her parents, she felt distanced, with no expectations of receiving anything from them. Despite their ostensible caring and willingness to help her, she rejected and acknowledged her aversion toward them.

It is likely that Joanne's sense of distance from her parents was reciprocated, especially by the mother, who talked about her daughter in a detached, objective manner. The father expressed more warmth, concern, and anger. This adolescent shared with adults who are diagnosed with PDs a history of lying, stealing since early childhood, and early sexual activity; narcissistic features of self-aggrandizement, self-entitlement, and aloofness; impulsivity (running away, failing to plan ahead); lack of remorse; and no friendships, no learning from experience, and no goals. Her inconsistent school performance, caused partly by a mild dyslexia, was rooted to a greater extent in her lack of motivation. Due to her impulsivity, her association with delinquent individuals, and her disregard for her own safety, the patient can be considered at risk for suicide or a severe accident.

DIFFERENTIAL DIAGNOSIS

Because *DSM-IV* does not specify the psychological characteristics of either conduct disorders or antisocial PD, it is important to differentiate antisocial behaviors in a variety of diagnostic syndromes from ASPD proper, or psychopathy (Frick et al. 1994), which includes both the traits of narcissistic PD and the array of delinquent antisocial behaviors.

In H. Cleckley's (1941) diagnosis, psychopathy is characterized by egocentricity, absence of guilt, superficial charm, shallow emotions, absence of empathy, absence of anxiety, and absence of lasting relationships. These are the very phenomena that distinguish children's milder socialized conduct disorders from ASPD proper (P. Kernberg and S. Chazan 1997). Children described as antisocial are unable to maintain social relations, are more aggressive, have less anxiety, and respond less well to treatment. Indeed, the less anxiety, the more severe the antisocial behavior, and the worse the prognosis (Frick et al. 1994).

As already noted, *DSM-IV* states that ASPD should not be diagnosed in patients under the age of 18; yet evidence of conduct disorder before the age of 15 is one of the key criteria.* T. E. Moffitt (1993) has shown that patients with antisocial PDs have indeed evidenced them since early childhood—in contrast to many adolescents who present antisocial behaviors only as teenagers. Many researchers agree on the two-faceted nature of ASPD, a narcissistic personality side and a delinquent behavioral side.

One way to distinguish ASPD proper, or psychopathy, is in terms of socialization. *DSM-III* identified different subtypes of conduct disorders: The nonsocialized aggressive, solitary aggressive, and undifferentiated types were included in the psychopathy group; the socialized conduct disorders, both aggressive and nonaggressive subtypes, encompassed the vast majority of the nonpsychopathic group. Aggressive socialized children manifest some capacity for peer relationships, attachment, guilt, shame, and remorse, whereas aggressive nonsocialized children are unable to understand rules or the feelings of others.

Because the two types have different outcomes, it is regrettable that *DSM-IV* does not take note of the important distinction between socialized and nonsocialized children. Socialized delinquents were more responsible on parole, whereas young offenders of the nonsocialized type were arrested as adults for violent crimes, including assault, rape, and murder. We may add that socialized antisocial youngsters get involved in antisocial behaviors to become part of a group, whereas the nonsocialized youngster does not show the motivation or capacity for affiliation, except for fleeting alliances with a gang in which ultimately each member is for himself.

In Frick and colleagues' (1995) study of 95 clinic referred children between the ages of 6 and 13, a similar finding of two dimensions emerged in the be-

---

*Because conduct disorder encompasses all the criteria for antisocial personality disorder as illustrated earlier, it turns out that to meet criteria for ASPD, you have to be an ASPD before age 18.

havior of children with conduct disorders. One was characterized by impulsivity and such conduct problems as delinquent behaviors; the other was associated with psychological traits subsumed under the heading of callous/unemotional, which captures such characteristics as lack of guilt, lack of empathy, and superficial charm. These two factors correspond to those described in adolescents by A. H. Smith and colleagues (1997) and in adults by R. D. Hare (1991).

Frick (1994) concluded that impulsivity and conduct problems correlate with low intelligence, poor school achievement, and anxiety, whereas the callous and unemotional component correlates with the sensation-seeking, self-aggrandizement, and lack of empathy that are congruent with narcissistic PD. These two independent factors, when linked with a higher level of intelligence, define the subgroups of psychopathy among conduct-disordered children.

To systematically assess the two factors in children and adolescents, both groups of researchers (Smith et al. 1997 with adolescents, and Frick et al. 1995 with children) adapted the psychopathy checklist scale (Hare 1991) to the developmental stage of the child. The outcomes provided strong evidence that ASPD proper, or psychopathy, can be found in adolescents and children. There are significant differences between adolescents who have phase-specific conduct disorders and those who have psychopathic conduct disorders. Given the more serious prognosis of the latter, differentiation is critical: Those adolescents who showed psychopathic ASPD, like adults, revealed severe narcissism, with less anxiety and more detachment; they also show lifetime chronicity (Moffitt 1993).

Loeber and Schmaling (1985) studied the differentiation between overt and covert antisocial behaviors. Their findings, in our opinion, are clinically relevant. Overt behaviors, such as arguing, hitting, yelling—that is, behaviors that reveal an emotional investment, albeit a negative one—were associated mainly with the panoply of oppositional behaviors, including screaming, impulsiveness, temper tantrums, and moodiness. By contrast, covert behaviors—that is, acts performed outside the monitoring of adults, such as lying, stealing, and vandalism—were associated with alcoholism, interaction with deviant peers, and truancy from school. This overt/covert dimension accounted for 69 percent of the variance in a metastudy of 11,000 children.

A study of 48 subjects aged 13 to 17 (Frick et al. 1995) using a modified Hare psychopathy checklist specific to the adolescent phase showed factors that correlated with narcissistic PD and antisocial PD, in keeping with the

DSM-IV definitions. The two factors were added, and a psychopathy range was established as follows: ratings of 29 or higher corresponded to psychopathic conduct disorder, 20 to 28 corresponded to moderate psychopathic conduct disorder, and less than 20 corresponded to non–psychopathic conduct disorder. The youngsters who scored 29 or higher all had a history of violence, with the majority having initiated problem behavior before age 10. Of the one-third of non–psychopathic conduct disorders in the study, there was a negative history of violence; the vast majority had shown conduct disorder after age 10. (The probability of error was less than .001.)

T. E. Moffitt (1993) studied the developmental course of antisocial behaviors in a population of male offenders. His analysis of the history of arrest in relation to age of onset of antisocial behaviors showed clearly that there were two types of antisocial behaviors, one that indicated a chronic life course of persistent antisocial behavior, and the other that was limited to adolescence. This differentiation is clinically relevant because it isolates psychopathy as a chronic personality characteristic, distinct from phase-specific adolescent ASPD who had conduct disorders as children, confirming the importance of that criterion for the diagnosis.

The behavior of conduct-disordered children ages 7 to 11 has greater power to predict adult problems with the law than behavior problems in the adolescent population. Indeed, three-quarters of adolescents who present phase-specific antisocial behaviors did not seem different from their preschool-onset antisocial peers. Preschool disobedience and aggressive behavior at age 3 manifest later as childhood conduct disorders and result in arrests by police in the early teen years (White et al. 1990). Because the adolescence-limited and the lifetime antisocial personality cannot be distinguished in adolescence, however, the two types are confounded in many studies.

Moffitt (1993) identifies some qualitative differences between them. For example, the types of offenses committed by the adolescence-limited group reflect a rebellion against authority and parental controls or the wish to attain adult privileges; they tend to cluster around vandalism, public disturbances, substance abuse, running away, and theft. The wide variety of offenses in the chronic type of antisocial behavior include victim-oriented crimes involving violence and murder; they are more likely to be committed by individuals acting alone.

Among adolescents with phase-specific antisocial behavior, crime decreases with opportunities for marriage and work. The vast majority tend to reintegrate into normal lifestyles because they have the flexibility to use such opportunities and do not have cumulative delinquent histories to haunt them; also, they are unimpaired in terms of social skills, academic achievement, and attachment. Chronic delinquents, in contrast, select jobs, spouses, and friends that support their antisocial lifestyle, reinforcing their antisociality or psychopathy.

The prevalence of severe chronic life-course antisocial disorders remains steady throughout the life cycle: 5 percent of preschoolers, 3–6 percent of 4- to 9-year-old boys, 3–6 percent of young adult males, and 4–5 percent in the general adult population. These statistics validate the hypothesis of the existence of a chronic antisocial life course; the uniformity of the prevalence rate validates the contention that ASPD is consistently preceded by conduct disorder in children. Police arrests of youngsters 7 to 11 years of age predict a life course of long-term offending. The forms the antisocial behaviors take will depend on circumstances and age, but the underlying personality organization tends to be maintained.

According to Moffitt, teenagers with phase-limited antisocial behavior do not seem to behave any differently from the persistent early starters in terms of frequency of law-breaking or general behavior. Therefore, a more specific clinical description is needed and will be proposed later in the chapter. Adolescent phase-specific antisocial behaviors can occur in other personality categories, including variations of the normal neurotic range of personalities, but in the case of the life-course persistent group, such behaviors will most likely be precursors to ASPD.

Farrington (1990) has shown that there is continuity in the psychopathic personality throughout life, up to age 69, despite a decrease in criminal behavior. The expressions of psychopathic traits are reflected in a person's history of abuse and exploitation and/or neglect of family members—that is, in the narcissistic personality traits of the ASPD patient.

ETIOLOGY

T. E. Moffitt (1993) proposes a sequence of etiological factors that interweave with environmental elements to produce life-course persistent antisocial behavior. Among the possible causes are disruptions in the embryogenesis of the fetal brain, prenatal factors related to maternal drug abuse, and perinatal deficits related to nutrition. The neuropsychological deficits impact on receptive listening, reading, problem-solving, expressive speech, writing, and memory. Executive deficits correspond to what has been described as compartmental learning disability, which includes inattention and impulsivity. Typically, lack of affection, neglect, and abuse surround the early life.

B. H. Price and colleagues (1990) point to the influence of neuropsychological deficits on chronic antisocial behavior, in combination with Attention Deficit Disorder with hyperactivity (ADHD) and the conduct disorder that escalates into extreme antisocial behavior. In their study, boys aged 3 to 5 showed more than a standard deviation below their norm on the Bayley and McCarthy Tests of Motor Coordination and the Stanford Binet Test of Cognitive Performance. Increasingly, the cognitive, linguistic, and behavioral attributes of psychopaths are related to various deficits in the frontal lobe, specifically the orbital frontal cortex, the intramedial temporal cortex, and the cyngulum. Particular deficits may account for various inabilities of the psychopath to process or use language in its semantic meanings; use of language appears to be relatively superficial and subtle and more abstract meanings escape the psychopath (Intrator et al. 1997). Research on brain imaging may continue to clarify how psychopaths fail to appreciate the emotional implications of words, events, or experiences.

When antisocial behavior is already in the family, the child is in a deficit environment, according to T. E. Moffitt (1993). Constitutional predispositions and intergenerational transmission maintain the spiral. Moffitt mentions that the New Zealand Longitudinal Study found that children's neuropsychological deficits and family adversity impact significantly on aggressive confrontation with a victim or adversary. Similarly, genetic/adoption behavioral studies report the highest rates of criminal outcomes when foster or adoptive as well as biological parents are deviant (Mednick et al. 1984).

Secondary complications accrue and sustain pathological adjustment as the loss of opportunities leads to chronicity. The failure to learn more adaptive social alternatives narrows the possibilities for change. This failure is poignantly illustrated by the psychopath's decoding the conventions of socialization only for the purpose of manipulating his way out of prison or treatment.

Comorbidity with learning disabilities, hyperactivity, and (later) mania, schizophrenia, drug and alcohol abuse, depression, and anxiety disorders complicates matters and entrenches chronicity.

Moffitt's contrast between the chronic antisocial pathway and the adolescence-limited antisocial behavior that seems to be phase-specific is supported by the fact that four-fifths of all males in the general population have had police contact for some minor or major infraction during their teenage years (Farrington et al. 1990). At age 13, adolescence—limited antisocial youngsters are in the wide majority; by the end of their twenties, three-fourths of them have reintegrated into the normal population. Because adolescence is often prolonged by convention (e.g., by extended education and by delayed onset of work-life and property-ownership) for up to 10 years beyond the attainment of sexual maturity, the time frame for adolescence-limited antisocial behavior can be considerable; moreover, Moffitt postulates a tendency to imitate the behavioral example of chronic antisocial peers because the lives of professional delinquents show more immediately tangible profits. (This view may go some distance toward explaining apparent social proclivities for delinquent behaviors—in other words, the increasing involvement in crime reported by Moffitt by sequential cohorts of male British adolescents observed in 1938, 1961, and 1983.) As adolescence-limited antisocial youngsters become young adults and as opportunities for jobs and commitments to others become accessible, they reenter the general population.

DEVELOPMENTAL PSYCHOPATHOLOGY

Behavioral problems of ASPD children are chronic, and they appear very early in infancy. Patients can surface as young as 2 years of age, when a child may be impulsive to the point of seeming driven and impervious to limit-setting for reward or punishment. Parents of such children suffer from authentic burn-out—that is, a genuine sense of exhaustion and being fed up rarely found in parents of other children. They may be quite devoted and involved yet experience a deep rejection by or distance from their youngsters. The parents may also experience real fear of the children. Indeed, in cases of psychotic children who destroy objects and can be physically threatening, it is not uncommon for parents to live with the chronic suspicion that their son or daughter may be stealthily planning to inflict serious injury on someone.

The father of one 11-year-old boy who fit the diagnosis of antisocial personality reported that one night he awoke to find his son by his bedside dangling a knife over his (the father's) face; the child said he was just kidding. The father was extremely distrustful of his son and never left him alone with his baby sister: The boy had already attempted to jump on her abdomen to make her burst "for fun." At the age of 3, his parents had found him setting fire to the living room.

The mother of a 17-year-old boy called during the psychiatric evaluation because she was missing a kitchen knife. The psychiatrist did not grasp at the time the seriousness of her apprehension until she learned from the newspaper that the boy had been arrested for murdering his neighbor, an elderly lady, with that same knife.

The absence of internal control combined with ruthlessness is quite different from what one encounters in the history of other children who also present difficulties in control but can express regret and genuine guilt.

The records and histories of these children denote a relative naiveté by a variety of professionals or responsible adults. Even in the face of information that seems clear and undeniable, a well-intentioned member of the staff will frequently imply that symptoms of behaviors known to be precursors of future difficulties (fire setting, cruelty to animals, deliberate aggression, intentional manipulation, deceit, lying and stealing) are somehow mitigated or reversible. So, even though psychological evaluation could indicate typical disturbances, the conclusion could be, "This child does not correspond to what is normally understood to be an antisocial child; he is changing, and he is capable of saying that he is desolated or dismayed by his behavior."

The putative improvement after two weeks in a new institution that was described in the foregoing case of Maggie is representative of just such a flavor of denial of pathology—be it due to wishful thinking on the part of the mental health professional or "honeymoon" behavior on the part of the "perfect" patient who can manipulate or exploit the clinical staff. The reluctance to diagnose persons under 18 with ASPD is certainly understandable because the label is a serious one to impose on children who are supposedly in the process of development. Yet these children continue to develop in a deviant way and will not overcome their problems. Their prognoses are guarded at best because a high frequency and high variety of antisocial acts in childhood are predictors of antisocial behavior (Farrington et al. 1990) in adulthood.

INTENTIONAL AGGRESSION

Intentional aggression in children is an early signal of the possibility of ASPD. Otherwise, one very seldom sees a child who deliberately plans to destroy and to hurt. In contrast with the borderline child who breaks furniture or hits his sister, for example, the quality of the aggression here is characteristically explosive and impulsive. Predatory behavior is planned, as in the case of the 3-year-old who would wait for his sister to put her hand in the door so that he could close it on her fingers.

The antisocial child plans her action to catch her victim unawares. During an evaluation of a youngster of superior intelligence, the child silently and surreptitiously took a plastic dart gun and aimed it at the examiner's face while the examiner was looking down and writing. When the examiner raised his head, he was staring down the barrel of the gun. The child said, "Don't take it so seriously, I was just kidding." To create this moment of terror, the child had to wait with the gun poised, silently, for some moments. The examiner experienced a chilling reaction to this highly unexpected moment, unlike any other, although he had tested many children. The discrepancy between the affect of the examiner and patient was striking. That is, the examiner felt it was a serious, frightening act, whereas the child said, "just kidding" with a sense of sadistic pleasure.

Torturing of pets is a frequent finding. One child put his three cats into a clothes dryer so that they would die of asphyxia; on another occasion, he pulled out a dog's nails one by one as the animal howled with pain. Here one can see the aggressive drive translated into deliberately destructive acts combined with sadistic excitement. M. Kruesi (1986), in a study of adult criminals who had committed multiple murders, found that all had tortured or killed small animals at some time during childhood.

The aggression of children with antisocial personality is typically expressed without investment. That is, the aggression is not triggered by rage or anger; rather, it is accompanied by indifference and withdrawal without positive affects. There are no overt neurovegetative signs in the behaviors, either in the child's appearance or in her language. The aggressivity is expressed in a calm form; destroying or killing in cold blood is characteristic. One adolescent murderer was so disconnected as his sentence was delivered by the judge that he was writing the grocery list for a party he was planning to have after the trial.

FRIENDSHIPS

Antisocial children have a particular way of establishing friendships. Like those with narcissistic PDs, they can be coercive, controlling, and nonempathic with their peers; they are also more ready to deceive them, exploit them, and drop them at the shortest notice as if they never meant anything.

Such children have unusually well-developed social skills, but their level of object-relations is well below their chronological age; their level of friendship is that of the 4-year-old.

A boy of 11 defined the friend who lived next door as identical to him; that is, he said, the friend was a liar like him and stole like him. He could not describe the friend's physical or psychological traits; he could describe him only in terms of his possessions.

> "Well, he is 11 years old. He has a water bed, a TV. Each time I go to his house, he has 4 or 5 other friends to play in his room." Doctor: "Can you describe Eric, your friend?" Patient: "Yes. Three bicycles, one moped, one BMX, transformers, G. I. Joe's."

A normal child at this age would already be capable of appreciating the company of others and would base his relationship on reciprocal exchanges; he would describe the personality of the friend with distinct features (Selman 1980).

Antisocial children do not have best friends or lasting friendships. They lose friends because of their exploitativeness, coercion, and lack of empathy as easily as they use their superficial social charm to develop them. They boast about having friends in the thousands, but they do not admit missing any one. Friends are nonspecific; one is interchangeable with another.

Some of these youngsters make friends exclusively with much older or even elderly adults who can give them undivided attention as well as opportunities for exploitation. For example, one 12-year-old who did not have any friends his own age, having alienated all the children in his school, spent his weekends in a nursing home. He said that his best friend was a woman of 79 and his second best friend a man of 84. When confronted with the possibility that they might not be around for too much longer, that he might lose them, he said that would be no problem: He would just exchange them for any of the other old people in the nursing home.

Finally, children with ASPD tend to associate with other deviant peers because their ruthless exploitation of normal peers interferes with real friendship development. It is not unusual for them to be chosen as leaders in groups because of their narcissistic traits—grandiosity, entitlement, and demonstration of absolute certainty in their communications. In unstructured group settings, however, they can undergo micropsychotic episodes.

IDENTIFICATIONS AND ATTACHMENT

The developmental histories of children with ASPD show their inability to bond with others, as evidenced by their fleeting and spurious connections with strangers and by the fluidity with which they replace one person with another. The histories likewise indicate profound interference with the capacity for attachment: They may, for example, have suffered from extreme neglect; some of these children as babies were left lying in their cribs for so long that their craniums are flattened. One child, reportedly unattached to his mother, would vomit the food each time she fed him; moreover, he seemed indifferent to her absences, would not cry when she left the house, and seemed to be more comfortable with any stranger than he was with her. This child's father had abandoned the family.

In evaluating patients in this population, it is important to inquire about their patterns of attachment to parents, siblings, and others because the quality of attachment reflects the parallel depth and specificity of internal working models or object-representations. At best, ASPD children have partial object-representations, such that they perceive other people in terms of their dependence on them ("She is nice to me"). More typically, however, there is a more primitive, ruthless connection whereby they relate to human beings as though they were inanimate objects. J. Noshpitz (1993) described an antisocial adolescent who said, "The life of somebody is like a balloon that one can make burst." This example illustrates both the ruthless nature of the aggressive drive focused on the physical destruction of the other person and the implicit devaluation of the internal representation of the other through transformation of an animate object-representation (a person) into an inanimate one (a balloon).

IDENTIFICATIONS AND THE SUPEREGO

The identifications of antisocial youngsters do not develop normally into the capacity to internalize the values and morals of their parents and societal norms. To explain their considerable capacity to echo and imitate other people nonetheless, D. Meltzer (1995) has coined the term *adhesive identifications*, denoting the superficial, short-term kind of identification that "peel off" and are not integrated into the ego or the superego. This distinction has practical implications for the treatment of children with ASPD because it makes sense of illusory behavioral improvements that only mean children have learned the rules of the game and are going through the motions. It may also explain the lack of a superego.

The concept of adhesive identifications may also shed light on the absence of a superego, which is constructed on the basis of multiple selective identifications with significant people from the pre-oedipal and oedipal periods, as E. Jacobson has described in *The Self and the Object World* (1964). In antisocial children, the identifications are superficial and do not fulfill the important function of forming part of the structure of the superego. Consequently, these children have no remorse and no guilt. They cannot conceive that there are people in this world who do not lie ("everybody, of course, lies"). Hence, they are impervious to reward and punishment (Farrington 1990). Moreover, they tend to see themselves as victims and to blame others for exposing them to temptation.

DIAGNOSTIC ASSESSMENT AND PSYCHOLOGICAL TESTING

During face-to-face interviews, antisocial youngsters are very polite and socially skillful, even engaging. Their veneer of instant charm is a trap for the mental health professional, as it serves to control and manipulate him and invade his physical and psychological space. Establishing the diagnosis should be expected to take at least several sessions—in other words, until the initial charm gives way to ruthlessness and omnipotent control upon the first occasion of even a minimal frustration.

STYLE OF COMMUNICATION

The affective quality of the language of ASPD children is dissociated from the formal content, so their discourse seems contrived, inauthentic, detached, and at times insipid. Speech flows fast and uninterruptedly, like a page from a James Joyce book, without paragraphs or punctuation marks. Words are used at least as much to deflect attention, to gloss things over, as for meaningful communication.

If a child acknowledges minor faults or misbehaviors, he characteristically omits or minimizes more serious problems. The 11-year-old whose father awoke to find him dangling a knife in his face acknowledged the incident to the therapist but left out any mention of the knife.

Antisocial children display an extraordinary capacity to guess the intentions and thoughts of the other; we have named this trait *cloning*. These children seem to calculate what the clinician wants to hear, and they imitate her attitudes in order to manipulate her. When confronted with these behaviors, they frequently react with a grin as if they love to be recognized playing the game of cloning.

COUNTERTRANSFERENCE REACTIONS

When so echoing the interviewer's thoughts, the ASPD patient can evoke the sense in the interviewer that he is meeting somebody just like himself. The illusion of intimacy thus created masks the real void in the child's emotional relatedness.

Such a child may elicit chilling reactions from the adult, either by direct threat or by the contents of their communication. An example is an 8-year-old who quietly said to the therapist in the presence of his mother, "I hate my brother so much that I would chop him into pieces, purée him, and give him to you to eat." Professionals and parents alike may allow the ASPD youngster to con them because of their wish and their need not to feel so frightened of him.

Antisocial children can attempt to establish an artificial and intrusive chumminess with an adult that blurs differences of age, role, or authority. For example, a boy began his first evaluation by commenting, "Oh, there is tea," and promptly serving himself. He also adressed the psychiatrist as a peer and not as being in a diagnostic interview with an adult, a psychiatrist he had never met before. In effect, he immediately took control of the situation; he appropriated the adult's desk and role, addressed the adult as equal, and used the room as if it were his own.

Whereas the narcissistic child may treat the adult disrespectfully, devalue him ("This is boring"), and challenge his authority, the antisocial child goes a step further by appropriating the adult's role and literally taking over the surroundings. With the narcissistic child, one might feel irritated and unappreciated, but with the antisocial child, the clinician feels controlled, invaded, and coerced. He can feel "taken" or "stolen from," so that he develops a heightened wariness or guardedness toward his patient. In interviews with these youngsters, it is not infrequent to have the feeling that the interviewer becomes the interviewee.

Moreover, the usual empathy experienced by the average clinician toward his patients is replaced by a sense of estrangement. Interviewing the antisocial child is like interviewing a hologram in the form of a person. The person can be recognized visually but cannot be touched because he is just made of air; there is no substance to him.

In that ASPD children have not only grandiose selves but also grandiose body selves, they feel entitled to expel gasses, swallow nasal mucous, and clean their nails in front of others as if all of these products were highly valuable. Also, their eating habits can be, as one mother said, "utterly disgusting."

DREAMS, DAYDREAMS, AND PSEUDO-INSIGHTS

The clinician assessing a 17-year-old who met the criteria for ASPD commented that "despite the fact that my patient is capable of admitting his feelings of suicide and homicide, he totally denied being able to put them into action"—yet he had already attacked another person with the intention of killing him, and the report indicated that he was upset that he felt no remorse.

Now, however, the patient was able to acknowledge his fear of losing control over his impulses. In describing a dream, he said, "I am cold. Nothing has an effect over me. I don't have a conscience. I don't have emotions. I am incapable of keeping anything inside of myself because they accumulate and then it explodes." His daydreams and nightmares carried the theme of killing others or making himself be killed by another person. In all of his communications, one could sense a certain capacity for insight. In spite of his revealing his awareness of not having a conscience, of lack of remorse, of not having emotions, of fear of losing control, he did not change his behavior. Insight without behavioral changes is called *pseudo-insight*. Indeed, a few days later, the patient stabbed an elderly lady, his neighbor, to death. Although his history and personality traits were consistent with ASPD criteria except for his not being 18 years old, he had not been considered a dangerous person. Yet the gap between his dreams and his actions had vanished.

A clinician in disbelief tends to minimize and/or deny information, and the patient learns to tell or to say what the clinician wishes to hear without assimilating the treatment. We have an 11-year-old who was admitted to the hospital, according to him, because he was a "bad boy," and the hospital was going to teach him how to become a good boy. He had already had one year of residential treatment and had learned to say the right words without necessarily changing his behavior. The substance of his insight was only the wisdom of parroting what he should say to manipulate his way out of trouble. In a hospital setting, such children show an uncanny ability to second-guess the staff.

PSYCHOLOGICAL TESTING

The WISC-R Test Profile for children with antisocial personality has been summarized by N. P. Rygaard (1998). These children score lower in the verbal section than in performance sections. They score relatively high in comprehension, similarities, picture completion, and picture arrangement and relatively low in arithmetic, digit span, block design, and coding. There are difficulties involving emotional meaning of words, changing strategies, seeing a problem from more than one angle, and understanding proportions and connections among elements.

The subjective world of the psychopath as seen through the Rorschach Test reflects his lack of attachment and covariant lower-than-normal anxiety. There is only a very weak measure of aggression or violence—partly because the patient has figured out how to disguise his responses, and partly because his aggression is so consistently discharged that he does not have to represent it. Sadomasochism is measurable in affective form, however: The subject expresses aggressive responses and pleasurable affect concomitantly. This measure differentiates psychopathic from nonpsychopathic personality: The response parallels the quality of the play of antisocial children, whose only moments of positive affect surface during their sadistic smothering or cutting of toys or figures. ASPD patients have a distorted sense of reality, and their defenses are typical of the borderline personality organization.

The Exner interpretation of the Rorschach Test reveals a significant lack of aggressivity and lack of movement responses in comparison with the normal population, which may be explained by the patient's easy discharge of aggression to the external environment and the absence of conflicts about aggression in her subjective experience as a result of her lack of moral values. One might add that the lack of positive or negative investment in others contributes to the absence of aggressive affects because affects are not issued interactively.

The egocentricity scale of the Rorschach Test yields a higher score, indicating nonaffiliation with others; the associated trend toward more reflection responses in atypical cards points to a greater degree of grandiosity. Significantly, conduct-disordered adolescents produce a paucity of texture responses that connects with their problematic attachments and corresponding poverty of affectional relatedness. The decrease in diffuse texture responses correlates with the absence of need for closeness with others, a trait characteristic of psychopathic adolescents, who tend to remain more distant from adults than do their nonpsychopathic peers. The latter, in fact, experience a positive need for closeness (Smith et al. 1997).

Conduct-disordered children of a solitary aggressive type constitute a subgroup that correlates with psychopathic personalities. They show in the Exner system a high-lambda, which refers to the portion of pure, simplistic form responses item by item. These children need to steer clear of complexity in their environment; they stick to the obvious and typically take a trial-and-error approach to problem-solving. There is avoidance of affects in others and a greater propensity in the self toward emotional explosiveness, measured by pure color responses. Less anxious than normal and chronically emotionally detached, this population manifests shallow affect and an atypical acting-out defensive style.

Formal thought disorders, perceptual distortions, and impaired reality testing are all deficits masked by the behavior problems. A perception of other human beings as uncooperative and not nurturing is characteristic of the antisocial person throughout his life. A high egocentricity index reflects the children's estrangement from the environment, yet grandiosity is not as evident in children as in adolescents and adults. This factor needs further study as differentiation of infantile and pathological narcissism becomes better understood (P. Kernberg 1989).

Some of these same measures persist in adolescents, such as concreteness, detachment, and minimal anxiety; incidences of chronic anger emerge, and cognitive improvements surface, although impaired reality testing and formal thought disorder persist also. The adolescent's Rorschach Test is devoid of whole human responses and empty of aggression responses; high egocentricity ratio and the increase in reflection responses show a growth in pathological narcissism. Thus, the two-faceted antisocial PD proposed by R. D. Hare is validated. Affective or mood disorders are more prevalent in girls than in boys.

TREATMENT

The treatment of antisocial personality disorders in children and adolescents is still in flux. In discussing severely disruptive conduct disorders, T. Achenbach (1988) contends that the prognosis is extremely guarded regardless of treatment modality. Certain treatment measures can be taken to limit secondary damage to the individual, her family, and society, however.

It is important to target those pharmacologically treatable symptoms that are known to exacerbate the psychopathic behavior—ADHD, impulse-ridden behaviors, and psychotic episodes. (ASPD patients who suffer from characterological depression are not as responsive to antidepressants as patients who suffer from mood disorder.) The family should be informed about the prognosis for antisocial personality disturbance so that necessary measures can be taken to prevent physical abuse of siblings, homicidal threats to parents, theft of household property, and general exploitation of the family. In some cases, a residential setting may be called for to protect the patient from suicide and to protect others from his violent behavior.

FAMILY INTERVENTIONS

The parents of younger children who meet the criteria for psychopathy and ASPD in childhood need very intense support in implementing special measures before they become overwhelmed by anger and hopelessness, attitudes that will only make the child more depressed and anxious and will elicit more antisocial behaviors. Mother and father must maintain a common front.

In putting these measures into practice, mother and father must work together and support each other. Both need to be aware of the victimizing child's propensity to assume and to exploit the "poor me" position, even though usually one parent or the other wants to give in to a soft spot that entertains denial of the seriousness of the problems—especially when the child evidences fleeting moments of regret or depression.

The measures outlined below are intended to enable the parents to respond to the child's weaknesses—namely, his lack of impulse control, conscience, and empathy—with the firm and consistent setting of limits. Parents must be encouraged not to act out their anger against the child. Communications must be issued with authority and expressiveness of content and attitude, and they must be directed only where the behavior occurs and by the adult involved (even if it is neither mother nor father but, say, a grandparent). Parents tend to experience grief and even guilt as they put into practice approaches aimed at protecting the family. Both sets of feelings should be addressed on an ongoing basis so that the structure of the setting as well as the specific interventions can impact the behavior and also the internal world of the child.

Sibling abuse. Given the proclivity for fighting and sadistic behavior that characterizes the ASPD child, the family should commit to a goal of no contact between her and her siblings unless or until she can interact nonaggressively. If problems arise, regardless of whether or not the patient is the initiator of the fight, parents are to assume that she is the one responsible and automatically take the side of the non-ASPD sibling.* This measure is aimed at enhancing the awareness, attention, and caution the patient must pay to monitoring her contributions to, and provocations of, negative behavior in others. Finally, parents should be guided by their intuition and not leave younger siblings alone with the patient.

Stealing. The immediate response to stealing must be to return what the child has stolen to its owner, in the presence of the child and, if possible, in front of the child's peers so that community reaction has a chance to impact on him and evoke a more powerful affective response than just "I am sorry." Return of, or reparation for, stolen, broken, or damaged items is to be made to the person from whom the items were stolen. If stolen money is already spent, a schedule for repayment, even at the rate of only a quarter per week, should be set up and adhered to until the debt is met. The adult should portray the theft as a matter of intense concern because the child's capacity to read subtle affects is very limited.

Lying. Given the ASPD child's propensity to lie and her superficial use of language, the parent can never ascertain the full truth. The child must therefore demonstrate behaviorally and by means of outcome whether, for example, she has done her homework or not.

Signs of repentance. The child must demonstrate repentance, not simply express it verbally. Because ASPD children learn to say "I'm sorry" in order to get rid of an issue, their apologies must be accompanied by corresponding behavior in order to be accepted. The adult should not be manipulated here by the assumption of the role of victim.

Contracting

The adolescent's exploitative ways may call for even more stringent approaches. For example, the lawyer mother of a 17-year-old boy spelled out a

---

*Time with siblings is to be adjusted according to the length of time that interactions without fights occur.

contract defining the parents' responsibilities toward him and the conditions under which they would pay for college and/or his maintenance.

> We will pay for college to the extent described below under the following conditions. (a) We mutually agree upon the choice of college. (b) You continue to meet at least the college's minimum academic standards to stay in academic standing as a full-time degree candidate. If you fail to meet such standards, we will no longer pay for college. For example, if you are withdrawn from the college, whether permanently or temporarily, for failure to pass or complete sufficient courses, we will no longer pay for college. To prove that you are continuing to meet the terms of this condition, you must arrange for the college to send your transcript to us directly. If we do not receive the transcript directly from the college, it will be treated as though you failed to meet the terms of this condition, and we will no longer pay for college.

In response to the son's irresponsible, impulsive spending on entertainment, telephone calls, substance abuse, and illegal drugs, the contract further spelled out specifically which college expenses the parents were going to cover and which they were not. And it continued:

> The following rules apply whenever you are at home: (a) You will not be given the key to the house. Be sure to call home before coming to be sure someone is at home to let you in. You are not allowed to stay in the house without someone of our choosing present. (b) You are not to use our offices as your own.
>
> You can request to join us for family functions. If after the decision is made to allow you to attend you don't arrive punctually at the time and place we specify or you do not properly dress for the occasion or your manner or behavior is disturbing in any way to the family, you will not be allowed to attend the function, and in the case of disturbing behavior, you may be asked to leave the function.

The details of this contract reflect the years of exploitation, theft, and unpredictable and inconsistent behavior the boy had inflicted upon his family. Follow-up after three years revealed that the exploitation and threats to the family had ceased; the boy had dropped out of college and was living a marginal existence.

Play Therapy

In working with younger children, it is important to facilitate the channeling of aggressive and sadistic fantasies through play and drawings and to encourage the elaboration of aggression in the realm of fantasy while actively discouraging its expression in unacceptable aggressive behaviors toward friends, peers, or parents.

> Seven-year-old Herman was told that he had some talent for drawing, and he was asked to write a book with illustrations of interplanetary battles. The themes he had played out with his brother and the very fantasies he had shared with his mother became part of many volumes of adventures, each of them two or three pages long, and the therapist urged him to expand the narratives. Herman's play sessions came to resemble an interplanetary TV serial, with carefully arranged scenarios that occupied half the playroom, ending in massive destruction and multiple murders. Typically, Herman threatened to maim anybody who dared to touch his property and drew a warning poster on which he pasted a doll with a severed arm—although a flicker of concern emerged on one occasion, when Herman put away the toys so that "other children could play."

To improve the social skills of the ASPD child, a sibling can be engaged in peer, dual therapy. The sibling's explication of social clues will help the patient learn to play with another child—specifically learn to use play for reciprocal peer interaction in longer play narratives—and thus break through her isolation.

THE ISSUE OF CONSCIENCE

One of the goals of treatment is to rebuild the conscience, the superego, by means of intensive work with the parents to establish a consistent, corruption-free structure, and toward an attachment to the therapist in full awareness of the initial absence of a bond. The process can be painful and trying for everybody involved, particularly given the realities of parental burn-out and of the extreme sense of helplessness and hopelessness parents experience as to the effectiveness of their interactions.

The fact that children with ASPD do not benefit from rewards or punishments to correct and control their interactions and behaviors constitutes a special obstacle here. As a result, the attempt to construct a conscience or superego is an essential step in establishing internal monitoring for both punishment, in terms of shame and guilt, and rewards, in terms of narcissistic gratifications.

To the extent that the child is capable of understanding, he should be told that he has a problem—specifically, that he does not have a conscience—and that there will be an intensive attempt to help him acquire this missing part, which is as important as having a limb or eyesight. The metaphors used to explain the situation should be concrete and vivid, and the attitude serious and committed.

A first rule is to emphasize what the child does and not to focus on what she reports she has done or has not done. The typically endless and frequent discussions of whether or not the child is telling the truth lead to a mutual sense of despair, even hatred, because there is no rational mechanism for proof except to stay constantly at the child's side, which is clearly impossible; such doomed communications should be avoided absolutely.

An attitude of realistic hopefulness should be cultivated. In the therapist's contact with family and school, any positive change that begins to surface should not be acknowledged as such until the child has maintained the behavior consistently without relapse for several months. Indeed, changes should be regarded with a certain disbelief until then so as to motivate the child to persuade his parents that apparent decreases in stealing, lying, impulsive behavior, and destructiveness at school are in fact real.

Only when the interventions outlined are clearly established and ongoing can psychotherapy begin to deal in a more formal sense with the narcissistic aspects, the depression, the psychotic paranoid anxieties, and the sadistic components that accompany the antisocial personality traits.

INSTITUTIONAL TREATMENT

Long-term residential treatment and group therapy have not proven to be effective in ASPD cases because the child or adolescent psychopath learns the rules of the culture in order to use them for the purposes of deceiving and manipulating the staff. The 11-year-old boy who spent one year in an excellent residential facility after he attempted to murder his baby sister by jumping on her abdomen or smothering her expressed no acknowledgment, remorse, or regret about his behavior. When he told the interviewer that he was a "bad boy and wanted to be a good boy," his attitude was one of total aloofness and callousness.

Not only is the behavior of youngsters like him resistant to all the supportive, educational, social, and leisure resources of the institution, but it sabotages the treatment of other patients, encouraging the acting out of aggression. One 14-year-old, for example, convinced four or five other teenagers to follow him in running away from the inpatient unit and "play chicken" on a six-lane highway while crossing on the turn of the red light until he was eventually killed by a car.

One treatment model in an institutional setting has been designed to counter the tendency of patients to learn the culture of the hospital and tell staff what they want to hear (Berlin 1991). It was used with adolescent or young adult murderers, psychopathic inmates who were considered untreatable by any other approach, and took an anticontingent approach in which anything that the individual did during the day was followed by unexpected and unpredictable consequences. The inmate patient was only to relate to one staff person per shift; he was excluded from contact with other members of the staff. Interactions with this one staff person followed a written script that had no connection to what the patient was doing. (For example, if he was sitting quietly, he would be interrupted and sent to the isolation room; if he was plotting with others or taking drugs, that is, breaking the rules, he would be rewarded by a trip to the cafeteria.)

In the context of an unpredictable, confusing world, the patient became either increasingly anxious (although such patients usually lack anxiety), increasingly depressed (although such patients usually do not show overt affective moods), or disorganized. These symptoms made him increasingly dependent on the staff responsible for him. The conditions changed him from an inaccessible patient to a potentially treatable patient now suffering psychological discomfort.

This treatment is the only one that seems to have some rationale in terms of causing the structures of the antisocial personality to break down and offering the patient the chance to reorganize in a more adaptive manner. It would require a great deal of planning and staff-training in order to be carried out objectively and compassionately, however. Indeed, it would require the support and approval of family, and ethics and legal authorities before it could be carried out at all.

PROGNOSIS

The prognosis for psychopathic patients with life-course persistent antisocial behavior is extremely guarded. One can expect substance abuse, erratic employment, indebtedness, homelessness, drunk driving, violence including murder and sexual assault, multiple and unstable relationships, and domestic violence toward spouses and children. These patients abandon and neglect their families and present a high incidence of comorbidity and psychiatric illnesses; they have a high suicide risk as well.

The prognosis for antisocial adolescent girls is as poor as it is for antisocial adolescent boys. Contrary to the clinical belief that antisocial behavior is largely limited to the latter, there are not significant differences between boys and girls. In the general population, 7.5–9.5 percent of girls met the criteria for conduct disorder as compared to 8.6–12.2 percent of boys (Pajer 1998). Antisocial girls have a tenfold mortality rate, compared with boys' ten- to fourteenfold because their crimes aren't as violent as boys' crimes—in other words, burglary and assault, not the usual female crimes of shoplifting, drug use, and prostitution. Those girls with psychiatric comorbidity had the highest rates of adult criminality. The comorbidity includes depression, histrionic PD (which in half the cases also meets the criteria for antisocial PD), suicidal behavior, and pregnancy out of wedlock. Their lives are characterized by domestic violence and high use of social and medical services.

PART V
THE PSYCHOTIC
PERSONALITY ORGANIZATION

V.1

Introduction

The characteristics of the psychotic personality organization (O. Kernberg 1975, 1978) comprise the structure that underlies the known psychotic syndromes when they are in remission. The patient will not show overt hallucinations or delusions such that the diagnostician could access the elements to make the necessary evaluation but will exhibit bizarre behaviors, extreme constriction in interactions that betray a paranoid psychosis, or intense oppositional stances toward the interviewer that persist in a rigid way.

This cluster addresses the schizotypal, paranoid, and hypomanic personalities, which correspond to schizophrenia, paranoid psychosis, and manic-depressive psychosis. In the psychotic personality organization, as in the neurotic and borderline organizations, there exists a structure with specific characteristics in the areas of identity, defense mechanisms, and reality testing.

IDENTITY

Whereas the neurotic personality organization has identity integration and the borderline has identity diffusion, the psychotic personality organization has identity dispersal. There is no sense of a good or bad self-representation but rather a loss of "I" or sense of "me" as an agent. The self-representation can be fused with object-representation so that there are no boundaries between self and object; it may be even be confused with inanimate or intermediate objects, such as pets [e.g., the healthy child plays at being a cat, the psychotic child *is* being the cat].

DEFENSE MECHANISMS

The characteristic psychotic defense mechanisms are complex devices for coping with such typical psychotic anxieties as falling indefinitely and fear of emptying oneself out. Although the patient may resort to projective identification and denial, the more typical choices of the psychotic personality are:

- Autistic encapsulation, a form of extreme withdrawal
- Motor freezing, such as immobility
- Constriction of thought and affect consistent with the patient's tunnel view of his experience and of the world
- Dispersal of reality, whereby the patient can protect himself from the enemy by multiplying him into many small-size enemies
- Deanimation—turning the enemy into a nonthreatening entity
- Animation of inanimate objects in order to exercise total control

REALITY TESTING

The patient has lost his capacity for reality testing. Not only is he at the mercy of hallucinatory and delusional experiences, but he also cannot keep himself separate from others, cannot empathize with the reality of the interviewer, and cannot distinguish animate from inanimate objects (e.g., the patient may state that she is receiving orders from the computer on the therapist's desk).

V.2

Schizotypal, Paranoid, and Schizoid Personality Disorders

DEFINITION

DSM-IV groups schizotypal, paranoid, and schizoid personality disorders in Cluster A, which is sometimes referred to as the Odd or Eccentric Cluster. These PDs are distinguishable from others along two major dimensions: One highlights the patient's avoidance of others and his discomfort and inappropriate behavior when he must interact; the second describes his thought processes, which are more obviously idiosyncratic than their counterparts in other personality disorders.

The proper placement of schizoid disorders in a classification system is a function of emphasis and theoretical perspective. We include schizoid personality disorders in this chapter to be consistent with the *DSM-IV* classification for ease of discussion. Descriptively, the schizoid PD presents with features that bear a certain similarity to the schizotypal and paranoid disorders and this forms the basis for their *DSM-IV* classification. However, according to the structural organization of PD, the schizoid PD has the same structural characteristics as the borderline PD. These characteristics are identity diffusion, primitive defenses, and the capacity to maintain reality testing (O. Kernberg 1975).

The hypomanic personality disorder, in the structural organization, belongs within the psychotic grouping. Regarding hypomanic personality disorder in childhood, we propose that the relationship between hypomanic PD and bipolar disorder may be the same as the relationship that schizotypal PD holds to schizophrenia; namely, one in which the differences are primarily of severity (Caplan et al. 1990).

DSM-IV's diagnostic criteria for the adult form of each bear striking similarity to the qualities that describe the childhood analog. Indeed, in each case the disorder "may be first apparent in childhood and adolescence with solitariness, poor peer relationships, social anxiety, and underachievement in school" (pp. 636, 639, and 643); each can evoke "teasing." These features overlap with those common in children classified as having social phobias (Beidel and Turner 1997) and nonverbal learning disabilities (Rourke et al. 1986) as well as those with avoidant PD because they all evidence difficulty reading social cues and understanding interpersonal nuances.

DESCRIPTION

This whole set of PDs emphasizes the individual's severe problems and corresponding anguish in relating to others as core and enduring features. It is not simply that they are shy: Shyness is characteristic of many young children, tending to diminish with age. These patients demonstrate deficits in empathy, in role-taking and understanding the perspective of the other, and in being able to effectively engage in mutually satisfying and comfortable interactive play and communication with others. Their conversation and actions can be inappropriate, they often do not react positively or show pleasure when they are praised by adults or peers, or they may display these affects in an inappropriate or exaggerated manner.

Children and adolescents with paranoid and schizotypal PDs are also distinguished from individuals with other PDs by the quality of their thought processes and their unusual behavioral style. *DSM-IV* further identifies Paranoid Personality Disorder (PPD) and Schizotypal Personality Disorder (STPD) patients as characterized by "hypersensitivity, peculiar thoughts and language" and appearing to be "odd" or "eccentric" (pp. 636, 643); they evidence "idiosyncratic" and "bizarre" fantasies receptively.

It is necessary to differentiate these PDs from Asperger's Disorder, which is categorized by *DSM-IV* as a Pervasive Developmental Disorder marked by significant impairment in ability to relate to others by odd, stereotyped repetitive behaviors and by an exaggerated focus on one area of interest. Another important distinction appears to be adolescents with nonverbal learning disabilities, who are sometimes diagnosed with schizophrenic spectrum disorder (Rourke et al. 1986) because they may display odd qualities.

SCHIZOTYPAL PERSONALITY DISORDER

Schizotypal PD has become a subject of increasing research interest because family and adoptive studies report an association that suggests a familial and genetic relationship between it and schizophrenia. It is thought that STPD might provide a window for studying the impairments of schizophrenia without the blurring impact of severe psychotic symptoms and the mediations used to treat them (Raine et al. 1995).

This perspective would be consistent with P. E. Meehl's (1990) description of schizotaxia as an underlying neurological deficit or S. Mednick and colleagues' (1987) diathesis stress model that posits an underlying deficit or liability that can manifest as one of the schizophrenia spectrum disorders (e.g., STPD or schizophrenia itself), depending on other biological and environmental stressors.

Accordingly, STPD may be an indicator of a spectrum of disorders that includes suspiciousness and schizoid introversions; there is probably a link between STPD and chronic schizophrenia.

The risk of paranoid PD may not be elevated in families with STPD (Battaglia et al. 1995), but many who are diagnosed as schizoid in childhood develop STPD in adulthood (Ellison et al. 1998). Schizoid and schizotypal personality do share extreme social isolation; impaired empathic ability; difficulty understanding social rules; abnormalities of speech, thought, and communication; monotonous voice; mild thought disorder and loosening of associations or tangentiality; possible suspiciousness; and overvalued ideas (Ellison et al. 1998). Schizotypal features are stable over time (Squires-Wheeler et al. 1992), and STPD shows long-term stability on its own, indicating that it is a discrete disorder that does not automatically evolve into schizophrenia (McGlashan 1986).

K. Kendler and colleagues (1995) argue that schizotypal traits are not particular to schizophrenia but reflect a broader vulnerability to nonaffective psychoses. In a related manner, some report that STPD is more likely to materialize in children of parents who have an affective disorder (Squires-Wheeler et al. 1989).

CLASSIFICATION OF SYMPTOMS

Different systems have been proposed organizing schizotypal symptoms. E. Squires-Wheeler and colleagues (1997) distinguish *Positive* (Productive) features—suspiciousness, ideas of reference, odd beliefs, magical thinking, unusual perceptual experiences, circumstantial and tangential speech—from *Negative* (Deficit) features, such as constricted or inappropriate affect, odd behavior or appearance, poverty of speech, rarely experiencing strong emotions, indifference to praise or criticism, and no close relationships. They report that positive and negative symptoms can coexist in adults and that their subdivision of traits does not define homogeneous subgroups.

T. Widiger and colleagues (1986) subdivided schizotypal symptoms in another way: *Cognitive-Perceptual Distortions* include odd speech, ideas of reference, suspiciousness, magical thinking, and illusions; the *Interpersonal/ Deficit Dimension* includes social isolation, poor rapport, and hypersensitivity.

A. Bergman and colleagues (1998) add a third. The *Paranoid Dimension* includes magical thinking and illusions, and the *Interpersonal/Deficit Dimension* includes social isolation, odd speech, and poor rapport.

K. Kendler and colleagues (1995) used structured interviews to examine 25 schizotypal signs and symptoms in the Roscommon Family Study, an epidemiological study of mental illness in rural Western Ireland. A factor analysis of their interview findings led to the following groupings:

Negative Schizotypy—poor rapport, aloofness, coldness, guardedness, and odd behavior;

Positive Schizotypy—illusions, ideas of reference, illogical thinking, depersonalization, suspiciousness, recurrent suicidal threats;

Borderline Symptoms—inappropriate anger, affective instability, jealousy, impulsivity, and chronic boredom;

Social Dysfunction—general lack of motivation, occupational functioning below expectations;

Avoidant Symptoms—social isolation, social anxiety, and hypersensitivity;

Odd Speech—cognitive slippage and odd speech; and

Suspicious Behavior—hypervigilance and irritability.

MEASUREMENT OF SYMPTOMS

Z. Ellison and colleagues (1998) suggest that these traits are best measured in structured or semistructured interviews, in keeping with the conclusion of Kendler's (Kendler et al. 1995) study of adult STPD that self-reports in the absence of an interview will pick up only symptoms and will neglect the signs that determine negative schizotypy and social dysfunction.

With children, both semistructured interviewing and information from parents and teachers are necessary for an evaluation. They should be supplemented with psychological testing, which is necessary to assess the child's ability level, his profile of strengths and weaknesses for learning and academics, and his thought processes and sense of reality. Neuroimaging techniques are also indicated.

A. Bergman and colleagues (1998) report that verbal learning in adults was related to cognitive/perceptual distortions but not interpersonal deficits. The Squires-Wheeler group found that negative features were associated with measure of working memory, which is consistent with E. Walker and S. Gale's (1995) determination that frontal neural circuitry accounts for STPD and its negative symptoms. The authors believe that this system is activated earlier in development than limbic circuitry, which is responsible for the positive symptoms.

CHILDHOOD FEATURES

In a study of children between 6.9 and 13.4 years of age, those with STPD and schizophrenia had similar thought-disorder scores and higher scores than depressed and nondisordered children. (The parents of the depressed and schizophrenic spectrum–disordered children did not differ on a measure of thought disorder, Thompson et al. 1986.) J. Gartner and colleagues (1997) describe a 12-year-old boy with features of mania and STPD: Examining the various evaluations he received over time reveals a consistent symptom pattern of odd behaviors, magical thinking, poor empathy, belief in extrasensory perception, ritualistic repetitive behaviors, and cognitive slippage. Teacher reports from the beginning of the Danish High-Risk Study (Olin et al. 1997) confirm that children later diagnosed with STPD were seen as passive and socially unengaged, hypersensitive to criticism, and nervously reactive to events; they did not show social anxiety until adulthood. This research suggests that social anxiety develops as a consequence of the passivity and hypersensitivity that reduces children's socializing opportunities. Their particular traits may also render them ill-prepared to acquire behaviors for mastering the challenges of adulthood for sexuality, intimacy, job, and autonomy and separation.

Treatment

Children with schizotypal traits and deficits may be treated with group and individual psychotherapy. Exposure to social skills groups allows them to receive instruction and learn interpersonal behaviors in an interpersonal context. Individual psychotherapy can focus on efforts to improve their empathic understanding by intensely dealing with moment-to-moment events that occur during the therapist/child interactions. For some youngsters, individual psychotherapy may precede group work by instilling basic skills and reducing anxiety to prepare them for participating in the group. The purpose of both approaches is to help the individual to learn to cope better with contemporaneous social problems and to develop resources to preempt or mitigate later interactive difficulties. When children and adolescents with STPD also meet diagnostic criteria for depression and anxiety, those problems can be addressed pharmacologically while the psychotherapy continues to address the social and interpersonal elements.

R. Caplan and colleagues (1990) found that children with schizophrenia and STPD had high thought-disorder scores. They contend that the thought disorder is what leads to social impairment because it prevents patients from taking the listeners' needs into consideration. Therefore, careful assessment for disordered thinking is necessary; when identified, it too should become a target for treatment.

The treatment outcome for adults with STPD has not been promising. In one representative study (Mehlum et al. 1991), even intensive inpatient treatment in units specifically designed for individuals with PDs generated little improvement during hospitalization, none of the patients was self-supporting at follow-up, all continued to show poor social adjustment, and all had higher rehospitalization rates than other PD patients (except borderline).

Clinical Example

Marsha, now 18, was first brought to psychotherapy at the age of 4 years, 9 months, at the urging of her school principal. In school she was very shy, oppositional, and controlling. At the time of referral, she would go to the bathroom at school only if the teacher would tell her to and then take her, even despite an obvious need to go. Her behavior in class was variable. On "bad" days she was mute and withdrawn from peers and would sometimes crawl into a fetal position under her desk; she would comply with the teacher's requests—but only without talking to her. Teachers noted that she was not well-groomed, did not wear conventional girls' clothing, and wanted, in fact, to wear boys' underwear. Her classmates started to treat her differently or to avoid her.

Pregnancy and delivery had transpired without incident, and according to her parents, any developmental milestones were within normal range. The parents noted, however, that Marsha had difficulty learning to expectorate after brushing her teeth and learning to use a straw, and they reported that severe stubbornness emerged at 2 years of age. Marsha would not let her mother brush her hair, refused to wear the clothes selected for her, and was able to control the family with her oppositionalism such that plans would often revolve around how to get her to cooperate. She would not apologize if she did something wrong, and there were times when she would not talk at home. When she watched television, she would root for the bad guys. Marsha preferred blue clothes and boys' clothes and underwear "with a little pocket" (i.e., jockey shorts), and she would not wear a jacket to school. She had been a poor eater. There were no reported sleep difficulties.

One day at summer camp, Marsha acted like a dog, crawling and barking, and her counselors could not get her to stop. It was said that her father had behaved similarly as a child, when he was often withdrawn and rode alone on the subway. As an adult, he was a financially successful professional; however, his family was fearful of his anger. The mother was depressed, had crying spells, and would scream at her daughter, "I hate you, life would be better without you"; she would tell both of her children, "you kids are ruining my life." The patient's sister, who was 3 years older, would act like a substitute mother, sometimes talking for the patient and changing her diapers when she was younger; as an adolescent, her sister was cruelly critical of her, however.

In Marsha's first treatment, she presented as extremely shy, showed significant gaze avoidance, and produced minimal speech with the therapist. She was suspicious and acted in a wary manner distinguishable from that of other anxious children. She would agree to come to the consulting room with her mother but did not always need nor want her there; she also brought her two favorite stuffed animals and readily took to play therapy. Marsha enacted destructive, oral-aggressive, and rivalrous feelings, especially toward her mother, and could acknowledge interpretations of her

234 SCHIZOTYPAL, PARANOID, AND SCHIZOID PERSONALITY DISORDERS

wish to be the leader and replace her mother as well as her fear of being separate and without her. She became less resistant over time, allowing her hair to be groomed and willingly wearing and requesting gender-appropriate clothes, including dresses. She became more confident and relaxed during sessions and showed increased eye contact; she also became more verbal and often spoke in a loud, shrill voice. She even began to use the bathroom after sessions. The parents decided to terminate treatment when she showed improvement, although termination was not recommended.

Marsha returned to treatment two years later. The teachers now said she was doing just a little work, was withdrawn, and sat by herself as if she were scared; she might complete writing assignments but would not take tests or go beyond pure rote learning. She did try to have friends and to be part of the group: She would mainly stand alongside others and sometimes banter with classmates. Parents reported that she referred to one neighborhood child as a friend but rarely got together with her; they said Marsha did not seem to know how to interact. Again treatment was discontinued after some improvement.

Although she had never demonstrated her connection to the therapist or the treatment, Marsha expressed upset during this second phase that the first phase had ended when she had not wanted it to. This feature is one we have seen with other, similar children. Namely, they do not readily express emotions toward the therapist, perhaps because many of them are not sure how to do so in a manner that feels safe to them—but they are able to experience these feelings. Their unexpressed capacity for connection may explain why those around them are often unaware that they have such feelings. Children like Marsha, who present as rejecting of friendship can actually be sensitive to rejection or abandonment by others, and they and their families need to be helped to understand that. Therapists must appreciate it too; the countertransference can serve as an important cue to framing comments that center on increasing the child's empathic awareness of the impact of his behavior on another person. Then the child can begin to evaluate whether such an impact is the one he wants to have and to acquire some skills for creating a different one.

Marsha asked to meet with the therapist again when she was 12 years old, again invoking her therapeutic connection to him. She wanted to focus on the anxiety she was experiencing prior to her religious confirmation ceremony. She was more related than she had been in previous years, when at times she would not talk at all; now, she would discuss specifics about her anxiety. She eagerly participated in learning muscle relaxation and breathing techniques, and also in developing and practicing things she could say to herself to help her through the ceremony. In the event, she performed very nicely. Her interaction with peers on the occasion showed how she remained on the periphery of groups: She would follow the others around but really did not talk to them and did not seem to know what to do at times. She could mimic their behaviors but could not take initiative or engage in truly reciprocal activity.

At the age of 12 years, 10 months, Marsha was tested psychologically to provide information that would help in selecting a high school for her. The examiner noted that her interactions were characterized by the avoidance of eye contact and restricted verbalization. She was cooperative but never showed interest in the examiner or engaged in the most basic of social pleasantries. She was also a very passive problem-solver. She attained a Verbal IQ of 100 (50th percentile)—with her lowest score (16th percentile) coming on the Comprehensive subtest, a measure of social understanding—and a Performance IQ of 86 (18th percentile), with her lowest (2nd percentile) on Block Designs. Her adaptive style, as inferred from the tests, was to ward off closeness; she could be quite suspicious, often feeling that she was being watched or scrutinized.

Marsha was next heard from during the summer one year later. She had been acting strangely at camp, and her parents asked to have her evaluated because she had made suicidal comments. The patient said that she was feeling and acting weird and that she looked like she was on drugs but had not tried any; she denied any hallucinations and did not rate herself as particularly sad. However, she had cried for two days about the death of the rock musician, Kurt Cobain, and initially wanted to die to be with him but was not sure how to. By the time of the interview, the desire was occurring less often, perhaps once daily. She had been a fan of Kurt Cobain's group for three years and had hoped to marry him someday. Then she said she was foolish, and when asked why, she said because he was "unusual" because he "didn't shower." She had been showing inappropriate sexual interests toward much older male counselors and also described sexual thoughts and interests that were not appropriate; she said that the boys her age at camp were stupid. Camp officials saw her actions toward the older male counselors as inappropriately forward, and they were concerned that she did not seem to understand what they thought she was doing was wrong.

At 14, Marsha began individual psychotherapy with a female therapist. She also attended group psychotherapy. According to this therapist, she associated with "unusual" children but seemed "odd" even among them;

none had become a close friend, and all eventually rejected her. Marsha never felt it was because of anything she did. She still wanted to be reunited with Kurt Cobain but knew to "keep this under wraps." She dressed in "gothic" style, favoring a great deal of jewelry with ghoulish images (e.g., eyeballs, skulls) but had learned to discriminate as to when to wear it. She maintained a belief in witches and visiting cemeteries, was preoccupied with horror movies and Halloween, but no longer wanted to die. She now had a boyfriend. He was older than she but looked fourteen and was also described as strange; he had one friend and was a good student.

Her therapist said she no longer acted inappropriately toward her but reported that it is often hard to know which of her statements were true. Her treatment had focused on learning what is appropriate and on understanding how she alienates people.

Marsha used to bind her anxiety by latching on to some teachers in high school, but she was helped by Paxil. Her social phobia was improved by treatment with Prozac (for example, she began to eat in front of other people). She thinks of herself as introverted.

Marsha later entered psychotherapy with yet another female therapist and continued until age 18. This therapist described her as showing odd behaviors, a preoccupation with heterosexuality, and a poor understanding of why her behaviors are sometimes seen as inappropriate. However, Marsha has been able to find other youngsters who are also considered outcasts by the larger peer group and who share an interest in the occult, and she has a sustained commitment to having friends.

PARANOID PERSONALITY DISORDER

DSM-IV indicates that PPD "begins in early adulthood" (p. 634) but can appear in childhood with the solitary, socially anxious, underachieving, hypersensitive qualities attributed to the three PDs in Cluster A included in *DSM-IV*'s description of adults with paranoid PD.

DSM-IV requires that the individual satisfy four or more of the following diagnostic criteria:

- Suspects that others are exploiting or deceiving him
- Is preoccupied with unjustified doubts about the trustworthiness of friends or others

- Is reluctant to confide in others lest the information be used against him
- Reads hidden demeaning or threatening meanings into benign remarks or events
- Bears grudges and is unforgiving of insults
- Perceives attacks on his reputation that are not obvious to others and reacts angrily or counterattacks
- has recurrent suspicions regarding the fidelity of spouse or sexual partner.

Mark was referred for psychological testing by his school and for psychotherapy by the examiner at age 10. He had been having trouble reaching a reading level commensurate with his intelligence, yet his verbal IQ of 122 was Superior, and his Performance IQ of 104 was Average. His teachers and the school psychologist reported that he rarely spoke to them and would neither ask for help nor accept it. He did use the resource room but never completed assignments; he showed no motivation to improve and no concern about failure. Psychotherapy had not been helpful.

His parents were concerned because he had no friends. The boy participated in scouts and enjoyed working on the projects with his father, but he did not develop friendships there either; in psychotherapy, he described one neighborhood friend whom he rarely saw and of whom his parents did not approve. He was quiet in sessions, did not initiate conversation about personal matters or his inner life, and refused to respond to questions about them. He could acknowledge that it made him angry to discuss this material, but he could not say why.

He would bring along catalogs depicting various models (e.g., boats, airplanes) that he liked to build; he also brought catalogs from electrical supply companies. He had read them carefully and could talk about his grandiose plans, which focused on safety and protection, for using the products. Basically, he was interested in alarm systems and was coming up with new ways to ensure the safety of his entire neighborhood, not just his home; he constantly emphasized the dangers that were around. He developed complex ideas for the ideal home (alarm systems, a variety of gun locations, ambulances, helipads) that were projected in the most serious of tones, and he seemed to appreciate that these ideas were listened to respectfully.

Over time he began to articulate his rage at his mother and older sister, whom he always described as very cold and cruel. He spoke about his father

in a more positive way yet once expressed eagerness to be home early in order to protect his dog from him. (The father was returning after extended
medical treatment, and the boy was concerned that the dog would leap
toward him effusively, only to be rebuffed and then hurt for showing his
love and excitement.) The only time the boy ever fully relinquished the
mask of containment he generally tried to maintain was the day he
lamented his mother's dismissal of a much-beloved nanny, which he attributed to her jealousy of the fact that the boy loved her so much; on that occasion, he allowed himself to acknowledge his enduring pain and sadness
coupled with rage.

Mark was never willing to explore the reasons he did not do his schoolwork. He never directly admitted that the work was hard for him, but he
gave the impression that the narcissistic pain of his learning disability was
enormous. He showed little reaction to, or comfort from, the therapist's attempt to explain the learning disability, but he was surprised and pleased to
discover from the review of his psychological testing that he was, in fact, intelligent. He described murderous feelings toward his teachers, who he
thought were out to embarrass him rather than help him. He could discuss
in detail what he took as slights when they tried to work with him, and he
would not consider that there could be any other legitimate viewpoint.
However, in reaction to news reports of youngsters who killed their teachers
and their classmates, he said he would never do that kind of thing because
he really did not want to hurt anyone; he focused on his self-protective motives. He showed some improvement when his sister went away to college,
as though he were relieved of one enemy.

Consistent with *DSM-IV* criteria for paranoid personality disorder, this
child could never fully trust teachers, therapists, or classmates enough to let
himself get close to any of them; he maintained grudges, was very angry
and bitter, and could not imagine forgiving teachers, his mother, or his sister. He was very suspicious and felt himself to be in such danger that he devoted himself to developing plans to protect himself and unspecified others
against attacks; he also remained socially isolated. He seemed to feel affection toward the therapist and to experience some pleasure sitting alongside
him, sharing his various catalogs, but he could never let himself articulate
this pleasure. He would engage in some games with the therapist yet rarely
initiated them; he seemed to welcome being asked (even smiling slightly as
if to say, "what took you so long?"), and he seemed to enjoy playing but
again carefully controlled any expression of pleasure.

SCHIZOID PERSONALITY DISORDER

DSM-IV describes Schizoid Personality Disorder (SZPD) as a "pervasive pattern of detachment from social relationships and a restricted range of expression of emotions in interpersonal settings, beginning by early adulthood" (p. 641). Individuals with SZPD show little interest in intimacy, are indifferent about getting close to others, and do not seem to care whether they elicit approval or criticism. They can show constricted affect, appear cold and aloof, and have trouble expressing anger; when they permit themselves, however, they reveal that they have painful feelings, usually connected to their social difficulties. SZPD may co-occur with STPD, PPD, and avoidant PD.

S. Wolff (1991a, 1991b, Wolff et al. 1991) reported on a series of youngsters who were originally diagnosed with schizoid personality. Her clinical sample, which was mostly boys (4:1 ratio), showed normal to superior intelligence, but they were failing educationally and socially. They had five core clinical features: solitariness, especially among the boys; impaired empathy and emotional detachment; rigidity of mental set and the single-minded pursuit of special interests (inhibiting adaptation); increased sensitivity, with occasional paranoid ideas; and unusual or odd styles of communication, including overcommunicativeness, especially among the girls (Wolff 1991a, p. 615). More than half the subjects were outgoing, some were withdrawn and uncommunicative, and some had elective mutism. They could not conform socially, and when pressed to do so, they could disintegrate with weeping, rage, and aggression. Wolff's presentation predated description of Asperger's Disorder in the English literature and *DSM*'s typology of schizoid/schizotypal disorders.

The subjects were followed into adulthood. Of the 32 children who had been diagnosed as schizoid, 75 percent met the criteria for STPD and two developed schizophrenia. Their overall adjustment was slightly worse than that of others in the clinic, as they remained more solitary, lacking in empathy, and oversensitive, and they sustained odd styles of communicating and circumscribed interests. The children Wolff defined as schizoid were distinguished from control children mostly by their unusual fantasies, their special interests (including collections), and their being described as loners (although more than half were outgoing); they were more likely to have specific developmental delays affecting language rather than motor development.

Wolff's work emphasizes the difficulty in differentiating these children from those who might be diagnosed with STPD or Asperger's Disorder. Indeed, she states that many would have been diagnosed as schizotypal had *DSM-III* been available. The children in her sample had much higher intelligence than the levels typical of Asperger samples. Her struggle to distinguish SZPD patients from those with STPD or Asperger's Disorder confirms the *DSM-IV* observation that SZPD is infrequent in a clinical group. We believe that a structural personality assessment to determine the underlying personality organization and neuroimaging techniques could contribute to delineate these categories.

We have seen some youngsters who resemble Wolff's patients in certain ways. That is, they present features of Asperger's Disorder but show a higher level of intelligence than is usually ascribed to that syndrome. They would not be diagnosed with STPD, however, inasmuch as they do not show the characteristic quality of oddness in behavior, relatedness, or interests. Further, although they may not interact with other children in what would be considered a normal, related fashion, they are not actively avoided—precisely because they do not display extreme oddness yet they might be seen as different, even "nerdy."

To illustrate, we offer two cases.

One youngster seemed to fulfill criteria for Asperger's Disorder and also had schizoid qualities. He was referred for treatment as a first-grader, by which point he had already spent considerable time crying in school. Although there were no concerns about his academic or intellectual ability, he seemed constantly overwhelmed; like the other children we have cited, he scored much higher on the Verbal (110) than on the Performance (88) IQ test.

This boy did not interact with his peers and seemed uncertain as to how to participate in their games. He always sought to please his teacher, asked a lot of questions before acting, and was very much afraid of making mistakes. Highly reactive to bodily injury, he responded to the smallest bump with agony and fear that the injured part would fall off. He did not show the clumsiness associated with Asperger's Disorder and in fact was a decent athlete, but he did not like to participate in team sports or to display the requisite aggressive behavior.

When he began psychotherapy, he never looked at the therapist, did not want to engage in games, and could not sustain conversation comfortably. Instead, he preferred to bring in books that dealt with his obsessional interest in trains and were specific to an animated TV series; he wanted to read the books to the therapist or recite the programs, which he knew by heart. The treatment focused on concrete aspects of interpersonal behavior, such as shaking hands and making eye contact when entering and leaving, and it emphasized the impact on others of his ignoring their feelings because he wanted only to repeat his train stories.

It was decided that he should not randomly select stories to share with the therapist now but would choose those that related to his feelings. Accordingly, the content of his repetitive behavior was used as a metaphor in his sessions. This approach continued for almost two years, during which time he evidenced significant improvement, including a marked decline in depressive and anxious feelings and behavior. He was then able, at the therapist's suggestion, to set the memorized stories aside and to talk more about the real events of his life; he would even come in and ask questions about his problems and concerns—if still in his characteristic, stilted fashion. His voice was sometimes monotonic; more often, it had an unreal lilt to it, as though he were a character on one of his TV programs, and his exaggerated inflection seemed farther out of place because his facial expression remained fixed and did not match his voice.

He was able to develop a true attachment to, and positive feelings for, the therapist, and he articulated appropriate sentiments upon termination— again, however, with unreal inflection and a fixed look. He spoke in terms of an enduring attachment and wanted to preserve the option of reconnecting in the future should problems arise. He eagerly sought out and communicated with the small circle of friends he had marshaled, whose group activity came to revolve around particular computer games.

His parents (who had rejected recommendations for group therapy while he was in individual treatment) had him enter group psychotherapy on termination of his individual sessions because they were concerned that, although his functioning demonstrated significant improvement, he still had that unusual quality to his voice, which they hoped could be normalized.

A second boy showed similar features. Although he did not recite particular dialogue, at first he would only talk about computers. He was a brilliant youngster who had more than a 40-point difference between his Verbal (Superior) and Performance (low Average) IQ scores. His interest in computers lay not in playing action games; he was writing programs and developing his own Web page.

He, too, evidenced gaze avoidance, which improved beautifully over time when the therapist institutionalized social skills (shaking hands and looking at each other at the beginning and end of each session). When his single-minded interest in computers and its effect on his communication was pointed out, he switched to discussing cars. Over time, what might be called a "hatching" process took place, and he actually began to inquire about the therapist's interests.

This youngster had great difficulty doing his schoolwork and showed signs of an attention deficit disorder, but his parents refused to consider pharmacological treatment for many years. As he allowed himself greater expression of feeling, he came face-to-face with the narcissistic disappointment that, even though he was brilliant, he needed help to complete his homework—yet he could not and would not accept it. He did well on tests without studying, however, because he was so smart, and he moved from being an outcast to developing some friends with whom he competed in collecting then-popular advertisements. His competitive style was so single-minded that he did not permit himself play dates, but he did participate in sports leagues after school.

CONCLUSION

When one considers that *DSM-IV* describes a similar picture for childhood STPD, SZPD, and PPD, and that it overlaps with features displayed by children considered to have a nonverbal learning disability or avoidant PD, the urgency for early assessment and intervention cannot be overstated. Youngsters with deficits in relatedness along with hypersensitivity and oddness by elementary school can and should be supported in learning social skills to avert or at least to modify the serious problems they are at risk for developing. Appropriate interventions include individual and group psychotherapy and, when necessary, medication to target mood, anxiety, and attention deficit disorders. We are concerned that many of these children are described by parents, teachers, and sometimes pediatricians as just being shy, with the implicit and mistaken expectation that they will outgrow their behavior; intervention in adulthood for children who start out this way is generally ineffective.

Longitudinal studies suggest that, when appropriate interventions are in process, parents'expectations of a return to "normalcy" for children with Cluster A disorders need to be moderated. Indeed, most parents are quite pleased when they see their children developing some friendships, even around circumscribed interests, because they offer considerable satisfaction to the children while helping to foster their acquisition of interpersonal skills and their discovery of interpersonal pleasure.

In our experience, so many of the children who meet criteria for a Cluster A PD show a significant difference between their Verbal and Performance IQ scores—children we might diagnose as having PPD, STPD, and SZPD, as well as those with social phobia and a nonverbal learning disability. Although S. Weintraub and M. Mesulam (1983) identified patients whose right hemisphere neurological deficit was associated with the emblematic solitariness, difficulty interacting with others, "weirdness," and difficulty expressing emotions, we would not localize the operant deficit to the right hemisphere. Specifically, it is our opinion that the processes with which these children have difficulty also encompass frontal lobe dysfunction. The larger point is that there may be a neurological explanation that accounts for the features that all of these disorders share.

The youngsters in question here also evidence difficulty with figure drawings; some struggle as well with the cognitive operations B. Rourke (1989) identifies for children with nonverbal learning disabilities. Just as they may have trouble manipulating colored blocks on an intelligence test, they may have trouble manipulating visual images (e.g., playing roles) to see things from other perspectives; deficits of this order may also impair their formation of mental representations of self and other, including their concept of mind and intersubjectivity. These and such other aspects of their disability as clumsiness and sensory defensiveness call for evaluation by an occupational therapist. Each child will need long-term, multimodal treatment.

PART VI
SPECIAL ISSUES AND
RESEARCH IMPLICATIONS

VI.1

Special Issues and
Research Implications

In this final chapter, we shall address some of the factors that impinge on the expression of personality, maladaptive personality traits, and the severity of a personality disorder. Among these codetermining factors are culture, gender, and divorce.

Next we shall present the influence of the *DSM* system on the area of personality disorders in children and adolescents and the negative effect it has had in the field. By excluding the diagnosis from the clinical repertoire, it has reduced the practitioner's awareness of the very existence of PDs in children and adolescents; in consequence, it has effectively discouraged interest in research.

Areas of research will be delineated emphasizing the importance of adopting methodologies appropriate to the formulation of a true developmental psychopathology of PDs. We conclude by citing factors that facilitate optimal personality development and deter the emergence of personality disorders.

PERSONALITY DISORDERS AND CULTURE

Although culture surely contributes to the overt expression of personality organization (Alarcon et al. 1998), there is room for substantive research on every aspect of the relationship between the two. Does a culture-specific personality exist? We look forward to cross-cultural comparisons of child-rearing patterns and also to studies assessing the differential impact of such patterns in the development of personality.

The incidence of PDs across nations varies considerably, to some extent because methodologies in gathering and reporting data differ—which evokes yet another challenge for research. For just one example, compare the prevalence rate of 26 percent in Germany per the Manheim Cohort study (G. Reister and H. Schepank 1989) with the figure of 3.32 percent for the general population of Costa Rica (J. Mariategui 1970). Another example is that antisocial PD rates fluctuate on average of 3.3–3.6 percent in Los Angeles but 0.2–3 percent in Taiwan (W. M. Compton et al. 1991).

Of course, cultural factors can be pivotal to the treatment process, not only because they texture the background of patient and family across myriad clinical dimensions (i.e., the relationship of Catholic and Protestant religion to cognitive styles, quoted earlier in the chapter on hysterical personality, Gardner 1968), but also because the norms governed by ethnicity, history, and religion will influence choice of treatment modality and acceptance of treatment plan.

PERSONALITY DISORDERS AND GENDER

With the active exploration of PD in children still in its infancy, limited findings are available to document the impact of gender, although it appears to affect how certain PDs are manifested. P. Kernberg and colleagues (1997) observed that inpatient narcissistic male and female adolescents demonstrated gender-distinctive forms of narcissistic behavior: The female patients were more devaluing and aloof, whereas the male patients boasted more. Gender differences in specific Rorschach features have yet to be determined, however.

Gender may influence the development of PD at the level of susceptibility and at the level of expression. Certain PDs in adulthood are associated more with one sex than the other: Antisocial PD occurs more commonly in men; women are more likely to be diagnosed with self-defeating, borderline, and histrionic disorders (*DSM–IV*). Gender stereotyping in diagnosis requires caution, of course; indeed, some children with maladaptive personality symptoms may go undiagnosed because their behavior may be considered typical for either boys or girls. Further investigation is clearly wanting.

PERSONALITY DISORDERS AND DIVORCE

The importance of the relationship between divorce and PDs is manifold. First, PDs of various kinds in parents complicate the divorce process, not least because there is greater likelihood that parents so afflicted will involve their children in their struggles, especially in the case of dramatic, explosive disorders. In contrast to parents with neurotic personality organization, those with PDs tend to appear objective and able to allow their children autonomy; in actuality, however, their subjective experience of separation anxiety, their own sense of abandonment, and their difficulty in perceiving the children as nothing but extensions of themselves all make disentangling their issues from the child's issues arduous—not only for the professionals involved but also, much more so, for the children.

The intensity and chronicity of the parents' exchanges, particularly in that 10 percent described as high-conflict divorces (Johnston 1994), impinge variously on the child's development of pathological personality traits. The effects of divorce on personality development in children begins before the onset of the divorce itself: The child exists within a matrix of an impaired and faltering parental relationship that affects each parent's ability to navigate between his or her own needs and those of the child. Even in the early phases of development when the child does not yet have a verbal memory, witnessing fights and/or being their target will leave him with a predisposition to anxiety and mistrust.

J. S. Wallerstein (1983) reviewed the results of her 10-year follow-up study, which clearly revealed the long-term effects of the divorce process on children and their development. She concluded that it produces overburdened children who become responsible for either their parents' emotional stability or their own emotional (and sometimes physical) needs, or both. They display a wide range of symptomatic behavior including somatic complaints, sleep disturbance, fear of abandonment, disinterest, underachievement in school, suspiciousness, hyperalertness, and emotional constriction.

The degree of the impact on personality was reported by V. Roseby and colleagues and presented in 1995. Thirty-two children (ages 7 to 15) whose high- or severe-conflict divorce families had been ordered to undergo a 12-session assessment and intervention to help the parents protect their children from further distress, completed the Rorschach Test, among other tasks. None had been previously identified as needing mental health services, yet the Rorschach results, as well as the entire battery, suggested that they were time bombs: The maladaptive, inflexible, and enduring traits they evidenced signaled PDs in formation.

For J. Johnston (1994), it is the unstructured nature of the Rorschach Test that facilitates bypassing the usual defensiveness that these children learn to develop vis-à-vis adults; the test, thus, can function as a CAT scan of personality organization. The child's way of understanding herself and her interpersonal world can thus be reliably compared with normative samples (V. Roseby et al. 1995).

The effects of divorce on personality development have been systematically assessed by psychological testing using the Rorschach findings with the Exner Comprehensive Scoring System (1991). The Rorschach profiles paint a disturbing and chilling picture of children who are interpersonally inept and unable to manage the vicissitudes of relationships. They trust no one but themselves and expect others to have malevolent intention and motivation. These children appear to have given up on the possibility that relationships can be nurturing, and they prefer to remain on the social periphery, avoiding either close or aggressive relationships.

One father in the study, a man who had habitually beaten his wife and devalued her in front of his children, drew an idealized family relaxing on a tropical beach, whereas his 12-year-old son, given the same assignment, drew tiny stick figures in the corner of his paper. The father's enthralled expression was a contrast to the sad, empty look on his son's face; the boy did not exist for him. The traits observed in the Rorschach attest to the reactive development and consolidation of features that may serve to protect such children from further pain and distress: Feelings are avoided, the expectation that adults are caring figures is eliminated or diminished, and hypervigilance against further aggressive and maladaptive behavior is established. These traits prove to be costly to the child's adjustment to the world beyond the toxic environment of his home, however.

In the absence of active relationships with others whom they can trust, children like this are left relying on themselves. Their self-image is marred and inadequate. They try to deal with the world by using their own judgment, inflexibly disregarding the signals of their own feelings. Emotions are suspect and to be avoided. The children, consequently, constrict any expression of feelings and deprive themselves of the further emotional exchange with others so critical to healthy development. The affects they experience most easily are anger and alienation; they assert some sense of self by taking an oppositional stance. Their conclusions about themselves, others, and the situations they experience are distorted because their capacity to see and to think about the world accurately is impaired.

This ominous profile is significantly discrepant from any norm of expected personality development. The findings also indicate that the personality constellations are quite stable—in other words, that the children are not likely to feel any need to modify how they experience and handle the world regardless of how maladaptive and inflexible. Short-term interventions have little impact on their fundamental personality traits—including interpersonal relationships, impaired reality testing, constriction and avoidance of affect, poor self-image—that characterize schizotypal, avoidant, and borderline PDs.

Explanations in the literature focus on all periods: before, during, and after the actual crisis of divorce. High-conflict parents may themselves be suffering from undiagnosed PDs that have eroded their marital relationships over the years or have prompted regression in the face of stressors on the family systems. The divorce process and its aftermath may expose children to chronic tension, parental self-absorption or depression and reduced availability, and aggressive exchanges. Distortion of the parent/child relationship in the form of parental demands for loyalty and companionship or imposition on the child of the role of pawn or spy, pathologically colors her psychological development.

If the cycle is to be disrupted, it is crucial to assess and to monitor the long-term impact of divorce on personality development in children as well as the ramifications of their bringing compromised traits into adulthood and marriage.

LIMITATIONS OF *DSM-IV*

DSM AND PERSONALITY DISORDERS IN CHILDREN AND ADOLESCENTS

The *DSM-IV* presentation of PDs attempts to be atheoretical, and it has been criticized accordingly by some (e.g., Millon 1995). We share the critical stance because we believe that most, if not all, research and clinical work related to personality development and personality disorders has an implicit theoretical perspective. Even in a purely statistical approach, the selectivity necessarily involved—data sources, measurement techniques, modes of analysis—presupposes some assumptions with theoretical roots.

In the absence of a unifying theoretical perspective, the *DSM* may have discouraged the kind of systematic research that would integrate developmental periods and the transitions between them to enhance our understanding of how psychopathology arises. *DSM-IV* effectively ignores the childhood traits and behavior problems continuous with adult PDs (e.g., shyness with avoidant PD, aggression with antisocial PD, impulsivity with borderline PD). In sum, the *DSM* system is nondevelopmental. For example, the conduct disorders that are developmental precursors of antisocial PD are classified in separate Axes as though there were no relationship between them; disorders of attachment in childhood consistent with adult avoidant PD are similarly disconnected.

The *DSM-IV* position implies that childhood personality traits are unstable and that therefore the criterion of "pervasive and persistent" probably cannot be met—yet we do observe many cases where the maladaptive traits pervade and persist for more than a year (viz., P. Kernberg on narcissistic PDs, 1994, and Moffitt on antisocial PDs, 1993). The *DSM* taxonomy also evokes questions: If Axis II disorders reflect stable characteristics, then Attention Deficit Disorder—which is not an acute syndrome that readily appears or disappears but that does influence interpersonal patterns—might belong more appropriately here than on Axis I. Likewise, Oppositional Disorder (also Axis I), which can only occur in interactive contexts and strongly affects both interpersonal functioning and the sense of self and others, seems, in our opinion, misclassified.

DSM-IV does propose using the same criteria for adult and childhood disorders. It disavows the suggestion that they are distinguishable (p. 37); indeed, it says they may apply to children and adolescents in those relatively unusual instances in which the individual's particular maladaptive personality traits appear to be pervasive, persistent, and unlikely to be limited to a particular developmental state or an episode of an Axis I disorder. To diagnose a personality disorder under age 18, the features must have been present for at least one year (p. 631).

T. E. Moffitt's (1993) work on antisocial behavior may provide an instructive model for examining apparent instability in childhood disorders across time, by identifying two groups of adolescents who exhibit the behavior differently. In one, the antisocial pattern persists throughout their lives, both prior to and beyond adolescence; members of this group are more likely to manifest an ASPD in adulthood. In the other, which shows an increase in antisocial behavior in adolescence, the presentation is phase-limited. If the two groups had remained combined based on their seemingly similar, shared adolescent traits of antisocial behavior, a crucial distinction would have been missed.

By extension, rather than debating whether or not personality and PDs are stable, it might be more fruitful to determine if there are subgroups of children within each PD type who show personality disorder features in a stabler fashion that cuts across developmental levels, and others, also impaired in their self- and interpersonal functioning, who show a more time- or phase-limited disorder. The factors that determine and influence each form are important to identify because they will have obvious implications for treatment.

Diagnosis Criteria for Personality Disorders

The foregoing information indicates that there can be stability or coherence to many aspects of the child's functioning across time that correlate with the development of PD. Demonstrating developmental coherence provides a way to think about how to approach the establishment of diagnosis criteria for PDs in children and adolescents and about how to investigate their manifestation at different developmental levels.

DSM-IV does not define childhood PDs by specifying criteria separate from adult criteria. This approach has worked well for depression (Kovacs 1985a, 1985b, 1996), whose diagnostic history in children comprises an interesting model. The thinking that depression did not occur in youngsters (in part for theoretical reasons) was displaced first by the belief that depression in children could exist but that it would be masked (Cytryn 1974) and then by the view that adult criteria can indeed be applied (Carlson and Cantwell 1980, Kovacs 1996), although there do remain differences. (For example, depressed children often show much more irritability in place of depressed mood than depressed adults.)

Costa and McCrae (1998), using the Revised NEO Personality Inventory (NEO-PI-R), note that small changes may occur for some individuals after age 30, "but from the perspective of the child psychologist seeing a fixed endpoint, [personality] development appears to be essentially finished by age 30" (p. 148). They further note that

the study of development normally presupposes an understanding of the fully developed individual. In normative studies, adult structure dictates the variables that developmentalists must attend to. A theory of language acquisition, for example, must be able to account for the mastery of grammatical rules that competent adult speakers show. In studies of individual differences, *adult status is the ultimate criterion that developmental variables must predict* (p. 139, italics ours).

In effect, they assert that adult functioning should provide the gold standard.

The reference to language is of interest because language development can serve as a use of case in point. Dennis (1988), in her work on language development and brain injury, has argued that comparing language development in the brain-injured child to the brain-injured adult impeded for decades understanding about the relationship between language development and brain functioning. She contends that it is much more promising to compare brain-damaged children and their normally developing peers (p. 91). By implication, comparing personality-disordered children and personality-disordered adults might also have limited value. It is necessary to define normative personality functioning at different developmental periods in order to adequately evaluate youthful PDs.

DIRECTIONS FOR RESEARCH

The utility of the current literature on personality disorder research is restricted by several factors that limit integration of findings and obstruct clarification of the nature and course of childhood PDs. First, clinical researchers often fail to differentiate whether a behavioral trait is embedded in a consolidated personality structure or exists in isolation. Research on avoidant behavior in children, for example, does not assess the nature of the avoidance as part of an overall, entrenched pattern or as secondary to simple phobia, with other aspects of functioning intact.

The T. Achenbach Behavioral Symptom Checklist (1991) serves as an illustration; even though more than 50 percent of its items can correspond to PDs, researchers who eschew psychodynamic formulations and prefer to view pathological behavior as discrete, unrelated symptoms will conceptualize obsessive, self-defeating, and dependent manifestations accordingly and will neither assess nor address their insensitivity, inflexibility, duration, and context. This lack of differentiation produces results that may be incomplete, inaccurate, or misleading (e.g., the gulf between children who steal to win peer support and feel guilty about it and children who steal out of a chronic sense of emptiness, entitlement, and envy of others and show no remorse). The underlying function of the behavior is key to determining its diagnostic implications.

The inclusion of adolescents in an adult sample, without analysis of age differences, constitutes a second methodological problem in the research on PDs. Recognition of PD in teenagers is commendable (although their incorporation is often rooted in the need to expand a small sample pool), but grouping all ages together obviates the possibility of isolating characteristics particular to one. To test our proposal that PDs themselves undergo developmental changes with age, creating the capacity for discrete empirical analyses is vital.

Finally, many research reports fail to document the first time the diagnosis of PD was applied to a given subject. Indicating whether the behaviors were noted prior to adolescence is especially valuable in determining the course of PDs and also in corroborating the ideas, observations, and findings of other investigators. We hope that those put forth here will elucidate the very concept of PD in children and lead to further, critical dialogue, research, and clinical awareness.

DEFENSE MECHANISMS AND ADAPTATION

Longitudinal studies are already yielding some basic results and pointing to further research activity. One of the first such projects has become a classic. G. Vaillant (1977) focused on how the concept of adaptation (i.e., adaptive ways of dealing with the environment and oneself) and the concept of defense are closely related. His study suggests that patterns of managing affect modulation and the kind of defense mechanisms and individual deploys will be pivotal to his adaptation over the course of his lifetime.

Vaillant classified defense mechanisms as Psychotic, Immature, Neurotic, and Mature. Individuals with mature defenses—humor, anticipation, suppression, sublimation, affiliation, identification—were the most successful in their careers, in their marriages, and as parents. They displayed the best overall social adjustment, closeness to their children, and capacity for human relationships. Their offspring showed significantly greater identification with parental achievement, more social success, a lower school dropout rate, and less incidence of serious delinquency and psychiatric hospitalization. Their parents even showed, in their forties and fifties, good physical health—in contrast to the third of the study group with the most immature defenses, who developed notably more chronic physical illness over time decade and a higher mortality rate.

CHANGING DEFENSES DURING THE LIFE CYCLE

Vaillant also looked at how personality styles, as seen through the prism of defense mechanisms, tended to shift during the life cycle. Whenever mature defenses increased between the ages of 30 and 35, neurotic and immature defenses decreased correspondingly. Also, fantasy and acting out diminished with age; sublimation increased proportionately. By contrast, men who remained perpetual "boys" and multiplied their neurotic defenses reduced their mature defenses during the same period; they skipped over the normative personality crisis of adolescent turmoil that seems to facilitate later development.

In Vaillant's study, isolated traumas seemed not to shape a child's future as much as an ongoing relationship with important people. In a related study (Vaillant et al. 1986), in which inner city boys both delinquent and nondelinquent were assessed 30 years later, Vaillant showed that primitive or image-distorting defense mechanisms like those typical of narcissistic and borderline personalities (splitting, denial, omnipotence, devaluation, primitive idealization) were acquired partly genetically but more importantly through interpersonal relationships. Chief influences on the maturity of an individual's defenses proved to be the level of social support and the availability of the father. Gender, social class, and culture did not seem to play roles by comparison.

H. Steiner and S. Feldman (1997) have pursued the element of adaptive styles as measured by coping and defensive mechanisms. The relevance of assessing this dimension has to do with the fact that such mechanisms do differentiate between normal and psychosomatically ill adolescent disorders, but they are also helpful in delineating subgroups of patients, treatment indications, and treatment outcome. J. C. Perry (1990) has formulated methodologies applicable to the diagnosis of defense mechanisms in adults, and P. F. Kernberg, S. Chazan, and L. Normandin (1998) have found it possible to assess clusters of defense mechanisms reliably in children at play.

Further study may be required to ascertain whether or not defense mechanisms are precursors of overt psychopathology (e.g., affective and anxiety disorders), as well as likely components of the psychopathology of PDs. The related question of resiliency—the capacity for adaptive and resourceful response to internal and external stresses—is another relevant clinical concept that could be objectified and applied with such an instrument as the Bond Defensive Style Questionnaire, a self-assessment tool promising for use with adolescents (Steiner and Felman 1995).

M. Lenzenweger and colleagues (1997) developed a methodology for longitudinal studies of PDs that permits cost reduction by means of preselection, whereby subjects who have first been screened as possible positives for PD are then interviewed by clinicians. Using the Personality Disorder Examination (PDE) created by Loranger and colleagues (1994), whose very strict criteria include behavior of at least five years' duration and manifestation before age 25, Lenzenweger found a prevalence of 6.74 percent for a definitive disorder and 11.1 percent for a probable disorder.

D. Becker, C. Grilo, and colleagues (1999) have pointed out the continuity of similar incidence of PDs in adolescent and adult populations. Dependent and passive-aggressive PDs were relatively more frequent among adolescents, most likely in keeping with characteristics of the developmental stage; the other PDs were distributed equally. The authors concluded that what was observed in adolescence is a valid form of PD.

FACTORS ENCOURAGING OPTIMAL
PERSONALITY DEVELOPMENT

Optimal development may imply not only a measure of normalcy, but in our changing environment, a measure of resilience. We have identified many things that can go awry in personality development: Given basic physical care and normal physiological maturation, the pivotal predictors of optimal development are a sense of safety and continuity of care by supportive adults. More critical than whether there is one caretaker or several are consistency and investment in a child's autonomy, acknowledgment of his individual characteristics and potential, and communication to him of cultural and ethical values.

The role of the primary caretakers—nuclear family, extended family, or community—is crucial, although the era of the computer will most likely change what is at this moment the standard. For now, at least, we need to facilitate and promote human links in a very active way because attachment leads to cooperation and an actualization of maximum potential and can thereby counteract destructive tendencies.

CONCLUSION

The research on PDs in adults has moved steadily forward, yielding new discoveries and highlighting new controversies, even reconciling some. The work on PDs in children has also seen controversies; regrettably, they have led to a pullback in research. Still clinicians continue to recognize the centrality of PDs in children, so the need for further work is apparent. Our perspective is that PDs in children, as in adults, are reliably identifiable and show a pattern of persistence that makes their impact pervasive and severe; they are also associated with other Axis I and Axis II disorders. Considering PDs in the diagnostic assessment of children can render psychosocial and psychopharmacological treatment more effective and constitute secondary prevention as well, saving the children and their families years of suffering and wasted opportunities.

References

Aarkrog, T. (1981). The borderline concept in childhood, adolescence and adulthood: Borderline adolescents in psychiatric treatment and five years later. *Acta Psychiat. Scand.* Suppl. 293, 1–300.

Abraham, K. (1920). Manifestations of female castration complex. In *Selected Papers on Psychoanalysis* (pp. 338–369). E. Jones, ed., D. Bryan and A. Strachey, trans. London: Hogarth Press.

Abrams, D. M. (1993). Pathological narcissism in an eight year old boy: An example of Bellak's TAT and CAT diagnostic system. *Psychoanalytic Psychology, 10*(4), 573–591.

Abse, W. (1974). Hysteria within the context of the family. *Journal of Operational Psychiatry, 6*, 31–42.

Achenbach, T., Howell, C., McConaughy, C., and Stanger, C. (1995). Six-year predictors of problems in a national sample of children and youth: I. Cross-informant Syndromes. *Journal of the American Academy of Child and Adolescent Psychiatry, 34*, 336–347.

Achenbach, T. M. (1991). Child behavior checklist for ages 4–18. *University of Vermont monographs of the society for research in child development 56* (3): 225.

Achenbach, T. (1988). Personal communication.

Ahadi, S., and Rothbart, M. (1994). Temperament, development, and the Big Five. In C. Halverson, Jr., G.

Ainsworth, M. (1973). The development of infant-mother attachment. In B. Caldwell and H. Ricciutti (eds.), *Review of Child Development Research, 3* (pp. 1–94). Chicago: University of Chicago Press.

Ainsworth, M. D. S., Blehar, M., Waters, E., and Wall, S. (1978). *Patterns of Attachment: A Psychological Study of the Strange Situation.* Hillsdale, N.J.: Lawrence Erlbaum.

Akhtar, S. (1992). Histrionic personality disorder. In *Broken Structures; Severe Personality Disorders and their Treatment,* Jason Aronson, Inc., pp. 250–260.

Akhtar, S., and Samuel, S. (1996). The concept of identity developmental origins, phenomenology, clinical relevance and measurement. *Harvard Review of Psychiatry,* 3(5): 254–267.

Alarcon, R. D., Foulkes, E., and Vakkur, M. (1998). *Clinical and conceptual interactions.* New York: John Wiley and Sons.

American Psychiatric Association. (1980). *Diagnostic and Statistical Manual of Mental Disorders, Third Edition*. Washington, D.C.: American Psychiatric Association.

American Psychiatric Association. (1994). *The Diagnostic and Statistical Manual of Mental Disorders, Fourth Edition*. Washington, D.C.: American Psychiatric Association.

Andrews, G., Stewart, G., Allen, R., and Henderson, A. S. (1990). The genetics of six neurotic disorders: A twin study. *Journal of Affective Disorders, 19*, 23–29.

Andrulonis, P. A., et al. (1980). Organic brain dysfunction and the borderline syndrome. *Psychiatric Clinics of North America, 4*(1), 47–66.

Angleitner, A., and Ostendorf, F. (1994). Temperament and the big five factors of personality. In C. Halverson Jr., G. Kohnstamm, and R. Martin (eds.), *The Developing Structure of Temperament and Personality from Infancy to Adulthood* (pp. 69–90). Hillsdale, N.J.: Lawrence Erlbaum.

Archer, R. P., Ball, J. D., and Hunter, J. A. (1985). MMPI characteristics of borderline psychopathology in adolescent inpatients. *Journal of Personality Assessment, 49*(1): 47–55.

Bardenstein, K. (1998). The cracked mirror: Rorschach features of narcissistic character disorders in children. Submitted for publication.

Bardenstein, K. (1999). Rorschach Features of Narcissistic Children. Unpublished manuscript.

Bardenstein, K. (1994). Narcissistic character disorder in children: Rorschach features. Presented at *The Society for Personality Assessment Annual Meeting*. Chicago.

Barkley, R. (1997). Behavioral inhibition, sustained attention, and executive functions: Constructing a unifying theory of ADHD. *Psychological Bulletin, 121*(1), 65–94.

Battaglia, M., Bernardeschi, L., Franchini, L., Bellodi, L., and Smeraldi, E. (1995). A family study of schizotypal disorder. *Schizophrenia Bulletin, 21*, 33–45.

Becker, D., Grilo, C., Morey, L., Walker, M., Edell, W., and McGlashan, T. (1999). Applicability of personality disorder criteria to hospitalized adolescents: Evaluation of internal consistency and criterion overlap. *Journal of the American Academy of Child and Adolescent Psychiatry 38*, 200–205.

Beidel, D., and Turner, S. (1997). *Shy Children, Phobic Adults*. Washington, D.C.: American Psychological Association.

Bemporad, J., et al. (1982). Borderline syndromes in childhood: Criteria for diagnosis. *American Journal of Psychiatry 139*(5), 596–602.

Benjamin, S. L. (1993). Histrionic personality disorder. In *Interpersonal Diagnosis and Treatment of Personality Disorders* (pp. 163–190) by Lorna Smith Benjamin. New York: Guilford Press.

Benoit, D., and Parker, K. C. H. (1994). Stability and transmissions of attachment across three generations. *Child Development, 65*, 1444–1456.

Bentivegna, S. W., Ward, L. B., and Bentivegna, N. P. (1985). Study of diagnostic profile of the borderline syndrome in childhood and trends in treatment outcome. *Child Psychiatry and Human Development 15*(3): 198–205.

Beres, D. (1969). Character formation. In S. Lorand and H. Schneer (eds.), *Adolescent: Psychoanalytic Approach to Problems and Therapy* (pp. 1–9). New York: Delta Books.

Berg, M. (1983). Borderline psychopathology as displayed on psychological tests. *Journal of Personality Assesment 47*, 120–133.

Bergman, A., Harvey, P., Roitman, S., Mohs, R., Marder, D., Silverman, J., and Siever, L. (1998). Verbal learning and memory in schizotypal personality disorder. *Schizophrenia Bulletin, 24*, 635–641.

Berkowitz, D. A., et al. (1974). Family contributions to narcissistic disturbances in adolescents. *Independent Review of Psychoanalysis, 1*, 353–362.

Bernstein, D., Cohen, P., Skodol, A., Begirgamain, S., and Brooks, J. (1996). Childhood antecedents of adolescent personality disorders. *American Journal of Psychiatry, 153*(7), 907–913.

Bernstein, D., Cohen, P., Velez, N., Schwab-Stone, M., Siever, L, and Shinsato, L. (1993). Prevalence and stability of the *DSM-III* personality disorders in a community-based survey of adolescents. *American Journal of Psychiatry, 150*, 1237–1243.

Bernstein, D. P., Cohen, P., Skodal, A., Bezirganian, S., and Brook, J. S. (1996). Childhood antecedents of adolescent personality disorders. *Psychiatry, 153*, 7.

Bezirganian, S., Cohen, P., and Brook, J. S. (1993). Impact of mother-child interaction on the development of borderline personality disorder. *American Journal of Psychiatry, 150*, 12.

Biederman, J., and Lapeyk, F. V. (1992). Comorbidity of diagnosis in attention deficit hyperactive disorder. In Weiss (Ed.), *Child and Adolescent psychiatric clinics of north America: Attention deficit hyperactivity disorder*, 335–360.

Black, B., and Uhde, T. (1995). Psychiatric characteristics of children with selective mutism: A pilot study. *Journal of the American Academy of Child and Adolescent Psychiatry, 34*(7), 907–913.

Blacker, K. H., and Tupin, J. P. (1977). Hysteria and hysterical structures: Developmental and social theories. In M. J. Horowitz (ed.), *Hysterical Personality* (pp. 97–140). New York: Jason Aronson.

Blacker, K. H., and Tupin, J. P. (1991). Hysteria and hysterical structures: Developmental and social theories. In M. J. Horowitz (ed.), *Hysterical Personality Style and the Histrionic Personality Disorders* (pp. 17–66). New York: Jason Aronson.

Blasi, A., and Glodis, K. (1995). The development of identity: A critical analysis from the perspective of the self as subject. *Developmental Review, 15*(4), 404–433.

Blatt, S., and Ritzler, B. (1974). Thought disorder and boundary disturbance in psychosis. *Journal of Consulting and Clinical Psychology 42*, 370–381.

Bleiberg, E. (1984). Narcissistic disorders in children. *Bulletin of the Menninger Clinic, 48*, 501–517.

Bleiberg, E. (1994). Borderline disorders in children and adolescents: The concept, the diagnosis, and the controversies. *Bulletin of the Menninger Clinic, 58*, 169–196.

Block, J. (1993). Studying personality the long way. In D. Funder, R. D. Parke, C. Tomlinson-Keasey, and K. Widaman (eds.), *Studying Lives Through Time: Personality and Development* (pp. 9–44). Washington, D.C.: American Psychological Association.

Bloom, B. (1964). *Stability and Change in Human Characteristics*. New York: John Wiley.

Blos, P. (1967). The second individuation process of adolescence. *The Psychoanalytic Study of the Child, 22*, 162–186.

Blotcky, A. D. (1984). Early use of the Rorschach in anticipating the transference of borderline adolescents. *Dynamic Psychotherapy, 2*(2), 157.

Blum, H. P. (1974) The borderline childhood of the Wolf Man. *Journal of the American Psychoanalytic Association 22:* 721–742.

Bond, M., and St. Gardner, C. (1983). Empirical study of self rated defense styles. *Archives of General Psychiatry, 40,* 333–338.

Bowlby, J. (1969). *Attachment.* New York: Basic Books.

Brazelton, B. (1973). Clinics in developmental medicine, 50: Neonatal behavioral assessment scale. In *Spatics International Medical Publications.* Philadelphia: J. B. Lippincott.

Brent, D., Johnson, B., Perper, J., Connolly, J., Bridge, J., Bartle, S., and Rather, C. (1994). Personality disorder, personality traits, impulsive violence, and completed suicide in adolescents. *Journal of the American Academy of Child and Adolescent Psychiatry, 33*(8), 1080–1086.

Brent, D. A., Zelenak, J. P., Buckstein, O., and Brown, R. V. (1990). Reliability and validity of the structured interview for personality disorders in adolescents. *Journal of the American Academy of Child and Adolescent Psychiatry, 29*(3), 349–354.

Breton, J. J., Bergeron, L., Valla, P. P., Lepine, S., Hande, L., and Gaudet, N. (1995). Do children aged 9 through 11 years understand the DISC Version 2.25 Questions? *Journal of the American Academy of Child and Adolescent Psychiatry, 34,* 946–954.

Brim, O., and Kagan, J. (1980). *Constancy and Change in Human Development.* Cambridge: Harvard University Press.

Broussard, E. (1983). *Justin's Reflection.* (Videotape). Infant-Family Resource Program. Pittsburgh: University of Pittsburgh Graduate School of Public Health, Department of Health Services Administration.

Browne, A., and Finkelhor, D. (1986). Impact of child sexual abuse. *Psychological Bulletin, 99,* 66–77.

Campo, V. (1988). Some thoughts on in relation to the early structuring of character in children. In Lerner, H., and Lerner, P., (Eds.) *Primitive mental states and the Rorschach* (pp. 619–646). Madison: International Universities Press.

Caplan, R. (1994). Childhood schizophrenia assessment and treatment: A developmental approach. In F. Volkmar (ed.), *Child and Adolescent Psychiatric Clinics* (pp. 15–30). Philadelphia: W. B. Saunders.

Caplan, R., Perdue, S. Tanguay, P., and Fish, B. (1990). Formal thought disorder in childhood onset schizophrenia and schizotypal personality disorder. *Journal of Child Psychology and Psychiatry, 31,* 1103–1114.

Caplan, R., and Sherman, T. (1990). Thought disorder in the childhood psychoses. In B. Lahey and A. Kazdin (Eds.), *Advances in Clinical Child Psychology 13,* 175–206. New York: Plenum.

Carlson, G. A., and Cantwell, D. P. (1980). Unmasking masked depression in children and adolescents. *American Journal of Psychiatry 137,* 445–449.

Caspi, A., and Silva, P. (1995). Temperamental qualities at age three predict personality traits in young adulthood: Longitudinal evidence from a birth cohort. *Child Development, 66,* 486–498.

Caspi, A., and D. Bern. (1990). Personality continuity and change across the life course. In L. Pervin (ed.), *Handbook of Personality: Theory and Research* (pp. 549–575). New York: Guilford.

Caspi, A., and Moffitt, T. (1995). The continuity of maladaptive behavior: From description to understanding in the study of antisocial behavior. In D. Cicchetti and D. Cohens (eds.), *Manual of Developmental Psychopathology* (pp. 472–511). New York: John Wiley.

Cavedini, P., Erzegovesi, S., Ronchi, P., and Bellodi, L. (1997). Predictive value of obsessive-compulsive personality disorder in antiobsessional pharmacological treatment. *European Neuropsychopharmacology, 7*, 45–49.

Cherbuliez, T., Fibel, B., Kernberg, P. F., and Selzer, M. A. (1985). Scales for rating PAJ. Unpublished manuscript.

Christenson, R. M., and Wilson, W. P. (1985). Assessing pathology in the separation-individuation process by an inventory: A preliminary report. *Journal of Nervous and Mental Disease 173*(9), 561–565.

Clark, D., and Bolton, D. (1985). Obsessive-Compulsive adolescents and their parents: A psychometric study. *Journal of Child Psychology and Psychiatry, 26*(2), 267–276.

Clekley, H. (1941). *The Mask of Sanity*. St. Louis: C. V. Mosby.

Cohen, P., Cohen, J., and Brook, J. (1993). An epidemiological study of disorders in late childhood and adolescence–II: Persistence of disorders. *Journal of Child Psychology and Psychiatry, 34*(6), 869–877.

Cohen, P., Cohen, J., Kasen, S., Velez, C., Hartmark, C., Johnson, J., Rojas, M., Brooks, J., and Strenning, E. (1993). Epidemiological study of disorders in late childhood and adolescence–I: Age- and gender-specific prevalence. *Journal of Child Psychology and Psychiatry, 34*(6), 851–867.

Compton, W. M., Helzer, J. E., Hwu, H. G., Yeh, E. K., McEvoy, L., Tipp, J. E., and Spitznagel, E. L. (1991). New methods in cross cultural psychiatry: Psychiatric illness in Taiwan and the United States. *American Jounral of Psychiatry 148*, 1697–1704.

Coren, H. Z., and Saldinger, J. S. (1967) Visual hallucinosis in children. A report of two cases. *The Psychoanalytic Study of the Child 22*: 331–356.

Costa, P., and McCrae, R. (1998). Personality in adulthood: A six-year longitudinal study of self-reports and spouse ratings on the NEO personality inventory. *Jounral of Personality and Social Psychology 54*, 853–863.

Costa, P., and McCrae, R. (1994). Stability and change in personality from adolescence through adulthood. In D. Funder, R. D. Parke, C. Tomlinson-Keasey, and K. Widaman (eds.), *Studying Lives Through Time: Personality and Development* (pp. 139–150). Washington, D.C.: American Psychological Association.

Costa, P., and Widiger, T. (1994). *Personality Disorders and the Five-Factor Model of Personality*. Washington, D.C.: American Psychological Association.

Costello, E., and Angold, A. (1995). Developmental epidemiology. In D. Cicchetti and D. Cohen, *Developmental Psychopathology, Volume 1* (pp. 23–56). New York: John Wiley.

CPQ Form A. (1975). Champaign, Ill.: Personality and Ability Testing.

Crumley, F. E. (1981). Adolescent suicide attempts and borderline personality disorder. *Southern Medical Journal 174*(5): 546–549.

Cytryn, L., and McKnew, D. (1972). Proposed classification of childhood depression. *American Journal of Psychiatry 129*, 149–155.

Cytryn, L., and McKnew, D. H., Jr. (1974). Factors influencing the changing clinical expression of the depressive process in children. *American Journal of Psychiatry 131*, 879–881.

Dahl, A. A. (1985). Borderline disorders: The validity of the diagnostic concept. *Psychiatric Developments, 2*, 109–152.

Davidson, R., Ekman, P., Saron, C. D. (1990). Approach-withdrawal and cerebral asymmetry: Emotional expression and brain physiology. *Journal of Pers. Soc. Psychology 58*: 330–341.

Dennis, M. (1988). Language and the young damaged brain. In T. Boll and B. Bryant (Eds.), *Clinical neurospychology and brain function: Research, Measurement and Practice*. Washington, D.C.: American Psychological Association, 85–124.

Derryberry, D., and Rothbart, M. (1997). Reactive and effortful processes in the organization of temperament. *Development and Psychopathology, 9*, 633–652.

Diaferia, G., Bianchi, I., Bianchi, M. L., Cavedini, P., Erzegovesi, S., and Bellodi, L. (1997). Relationship between obsessive-compulsive personality disorder and obsessive-compulsive disorder. *Comprehensive Psychiatry, 38*(1), 38–42.

Diagnostic Criteria from *DSM-IV*. (1994). Washington, D.C.: American Psychiatric Association, 280.

Digman, J. (1994). Child personality and temperament: Does the Five-Factor Model embrace both domains? In C. Halverson Jr., G. Kohnstamm, and R. Martin (eds.), *The Developing Structure of Temperament and Personality from Infancy to Adulthood* (pp. 323–338). Hillsdale, N.J.: Lawrence Erlbaum.

Dodge, K., Pettit, G., McClaskey, C., and Browne, M. (1986). Social competence in children. *Monographs of the Society for Research in Child Development, 51*(2), 1–85.

Dow, S., Sonies, B., Scheib, D., Moss, S., and Leonard, H. (1995). Practical guidelines for the assessment and treatment of selective mutism. *Journal of the American Academy of Child and Adolescent Psychiatry, 34*(7), 836–846.

Easser, B. R., and Lesser, S. R. (1965). Hysterical personality: A re-evaluation. *Psychoanalytic Quarterly, 34*, 390–405.

Eaton, W. (1994). Temperament, development, and the Five-Factor Model: Lessons from activity level. In C. Halverson Jr., G. Kohnstamm, and R. Martin (eds.), *The Developing Structure of Temperament and Personality from Infancy to Adulthood* (pp. 173–188). Hillsdale, N.J.: Lawrence Erlbaum.

Ebata, A., and Moos, R. (1994). Persoanl, situational and contextual correlates of coping in adolescence. *Journal of research on adolescents 4*: 99–125.

Egan, J., and Kernberg, P. F. (1984). Pathological narcissism in childhood. *Journal of the American Psychoanalytic Association, 32*(1), 39–62.

Ekstein, R., and Friedman, S. (1967). Object constancy and psychotic reconstruction. *Psychoanalytic Study of the Child, 22*, 357–374.

Ekstein, R., and Wallerstein, J. (1954) Observations on the psychology of borderline and psychotic children. *The Psychoanalytic Study of the Child 9*, 344–369.

Ellison, Z., van Os, J., and Murray, R. (1998). Special feature: Childhood personality characteristics of schizophrenia: Manifestations of, or risk factors for, the disorder? *Journal of Personality Disorder, 12*, 247–261.

Engel, M. (1963). Psychological testing of borderline psychotic children. *Archives of General Psychiatry, 8*(196), 426–434.

Erdberg, Philip (1996). Personal communication.

Erdberg, P. (1990). Rorschach assessment. In G. Goldstein and M. Hersen (Eds.), *Handbook of Psychological Assessment, 2nd Edition*. New York: Pergamon, 387–399.

Erickson, E. H. (1959). The theory of infantile sexuality. In *Childhood and Society* (pp. 42–92). New York: W. W. Norton.

Erikson, E. (1959). *Identity and the Life Cycle*. Psychological Issues Monograph I. New York: International Universities Press.

Erikson, E. (1968). *Identity: Youth and Crisis*. New York: W. W. Norton.

Erikson, E. H. (1959). Identity and the life cycle. *Psychological Issues 1*.

Exner, J. E., Jr. (1986). *The Rorschach: A Comprehensive System. Volume 1: Basic Foundations*. 2nd ed. New York: John Wiley.

Exner, J. E., Jr., and Weiner, I. B. (1982). *The Rorschach: A Comprehensive System. Volume 3: Assessment of Children and Adolescents*. New York: John Wiley.

Exner, J. E., Jr., and Weiner, I. B. (1995). *The Rorschach: A Comprehensive System. Volume 3: Assessment of Children and Adolescents*. 2nd ed. New York: John Wiley.

Farrington, D. P., Gallagher, B., Morley, L., St. Ledger, R. J., West, D. J., Magnusson, D., Bergman, L. (1990). *Data quality in longitudinal research*. New York: Cambridge University Press, 285.

Fenichel, O. (1945). *The Psychoanalytic Theory of the Neurosis*. New York: W. W. Norton.

Flament, M. F., Koby, E., Rapoport, J. L., Berg, C. J., Zahn, T., Cox, C., Denckla, M., and Lenane, M. (1990). Childhood obsessive-compulsive disorder: A prospective follow-up study. *Journal of Child Psychology and Psychiatry, 31*(3), 363–380.

Fonagy, P., and Target, M. (1997). Attachment and reflective function: Their role in self-organization. *Development and Psychopathology, 9*, 679–700.

Forth, A. E., Hart, S. D., and Hare, R. D. (1990). Assessment of psychopathy in male group offenders: Psychological assessment. *American Journal of Consulting and Clinical Psychology, 2*(3), 342–344.

Francis, G., and D'Elia, F. (1994). Avoidant disorder. In T. Ollendick, N. King, and William Yules (eds.), *International Handbook of Phobic and Anxiety Disorders in Children and Adolescents: Issues in Clinical Child Psychology* (pp. 131–143). New York: Plenum Press.

Francis, G., Last, C., and Strauss, C. (1992). Avoidant disorder and social phobia in children and adolescents. *Journal of the American Academy of Child and Adolescent Psychiatry, 31*(6), 1086–1089.

Freud, A. (1936). *The Ego and the Mechanisms of Defense (C. Baines Trans)*. London: Hogarth Press.

Freud, S. (1964). Analysis terminable and interminable. In J. Strachey (ed. and trans.), *The Standard Edition of the Complete Psychological Works of Sigmund Freud* (vol. 23, pp. 253–290). London: Hogarth Press. (Original work published 1937).

Frick, P. J., O'Brien, B. S., Wooton S. M., and McBurnett, K. C. (1994). Psychopathy and conduct problems in children. *Journal of Abnormal Psychology, 103,* 700–707.

Friedman, R., et al. (1982). *DSM-III* and affective pathology in hospitalized adolescents. *Journal of Nervous and Mental Disease, 170,* 511–521.

Frijling-Schreuder, E. C. M. (1969). Borderline states in children. *Psychoanalytic Study of the Child, 24,* 307–327.

Frosch, J. (1971). Techniques in regard to some specific ego deficits in the treatment of borderline patients. *Psychiatric Quarterly, 45,* 216–220.

Gabbard, G. O., and Coyne, L. (1987). Predictors of response of antisocial patients to hospital treatment. *Hospital and Community Psychiatry, 38,* 1181–1185.

Gardner, D. L., Lucas, P. B., and Cowdry, R. W. (1987). Soft sign neurological abnormalities in borderline personality disorder and normal control subjects. *Journal of Nervous and Mental Disease, 175,* 177–180.

Gardner, R., and A. Moriarty. (1968). Dimensions of cognitive control at preadolescence. In R. Gardner (ed.), *Personality Development at Preadolescence* (pp. 118–148). Seattle: University of Washington Press.

Gardner, R., Riley, W., and Moriarty, A. (1968). *Personality Development at Preadolescence: Exploration of Structure Formation.* Seattle: University of Washington Press.

Garfias, H. (1998). Carta Aerea. Editorial Los Andes.

Gartner, J., Weintraub, S., and Carlson, G. (1997). Childhood onset psychosis: Evolution and comorbidity. *American Journal of Psychiatry, 154,* 256–261.

Gartner, J., Hurt, S., and Gartner, A. (1989). Psychological test signs of borderline personality disorder: A review of the empirical literature. *Journal of Personality Assessment 53,* 423–441.

Geleerd, E. R. (1958). Borderline states in childhood and adolescence. *Psychoanalytic Study of the Child, 13,* 279–295.

Gjerde, P. (1993). Depressive symptoms in young adults: A developmental perspective on gender differences. In D. Funder, R. D. Parke, C. Tomlinson-Keasey, and K. Widaman (eds.), *Studying Lives Through Time: Personality and Development* (pp. 255–288). Washington, D.C.: American Psychological Association.

Goldberg, L., and Rosolack, T. (1994). The big five factor structure as an integrative framework: An empiricial comparison with Eysenck's P-E-N model. In C. Halverson Jr., G. Kohnstamm, and R. Martin (eds.), *The Developing Structure of Temperament and Personality from Infancy to Adulthood* (pp. 7–36). Hillsdale, N.J.: Lawrence Erlbaum.

Goldstein, M. (1997). Children with schizophrenia-spectrum disorders: Thought disorder and communication problems in a family interactional context. *Journal of Child Psychology and Psychiatry, 38,* 421–429.

Golombek, H., Marton, P., Stein, B., and Korenblum, M. (1986). Personality dysfunction and behavioral disturbances in early adolescence. *Journal of the American Academy of Child Psychiatry, 25,* 697–703.

Greenson, R. R. (1954). The struggle against identification. *Journal of the American Psychoanalytic Association, 2,* 200–217.

Grilo, C. M., McGlashan, T., Quinlain, D. M., Walker, M. L., Greenfeld, D., and Edell, W. (1998). Frequency of personality disorders in two age cohorts of psychiatric inpatients. *Amer. Journal of Psychiatry, 155,* 1.

Grinker. R. R., Sr., Werble, B., and Drye, R. C. (1968). *The borderline syndrome.* New York: Basic Books.

Gualtieri, C. T., Komath, U., and Bourgondien, M. E. (1983). *Journal of Autism and Developmental Disorders 13*: 1.

Gunderson, J. (1977). Characteristics of borderline. In P. Hartocollis (Ed.), *Borderline personality disorders: The concept, the syndrome, the patient.* New York: International Universities Press, 1977.

Gunderson, J., Ronningstam, E., and Bodkin, A. (1990). The diagnostic interview for narcissistic patients. *Archives of General Psychiatry, 47,* 676–680.

Hagekull, B. (1994). Infant temperament and early childhood functioning: Possible relations to the Five-Factor Model. In C. Halverson, Jr., G. Kohnstamm, and R. Martin (Eds.), *The developing structure of temperament and personality from infancy to adulthood,* 227–240. Hillsdale, N.J.: Erlbaum.

Hamilton, D., and King, N. (1991). Reliability of a behavioral avoidance test for the assessment of dog phobic children. *Psychological Reports, 69*(1), 18.

Hare, R. D. (1991). *The Hare Psychopathy Checklist—Revised (PCC—R).* Toronto: Multi-Health Systems.

Harpur, F. J., and Hare, R. D. (1991) The assessment of psychopathy as a function of age. Unpublished manuscript.

Harpur, T. S., Hare, R. D., and Hakstran, A. R. (1989). Two factor conceptualization of psychopathy: Construct validity and assessment implications. *Psychological Assessment, 1,* 6–17.

Harter, S., Yawkey, T. D., and Johnson, J. E. (1988). Integrative processes and socialization: Early to middle childhood. Hillsdale, N.J.: Lawrence Erlbaum Associates, 258.

Hartocollis, P. (1968). The syndrome of minimal brain dysfunction in young adult patients. *Bulletin of the Menninger Clinic 32* (2), 102–104.

Henn, F. A., Bardwell, R., and Jenkins, R. L. (1980). Juvenile delinquents. Revised. Adult Criminal Activity. *Archives of General Psychiatry, 37,* 1160–1163.

Hoffman, M. (1977). Empathy, its development and pre-social implications. *Nebraska Symposium on Motivation, 25,* 169–217.

Horowitz, M. J. (1977). The core characteristics of hysterical personality. In M. J. Horowitz (ed.), *Hysterical Personality* (pp. 3–6). New York: Jason Aronson.

Horowitz, M. J., Markman, H. C., Stinson, C. H., Fridhandler, B., and Ghannam, J. H. (1990). A classification theory of defense. In J. L. Singer (ed.), *Repression and Disso-*

ciation: Implications for Personality Theory, Psychopathology and Health (pp. 61–84). Chicago: University of Chicago Press.

Hurt, S., Clarkin, J., Munroe-Blum, H., and Marziali, E. (1992). Borderline behavioral clusters and different treatment approaches. In J. Clarkin, E. Marziali, and H. Munroe-Blum (eds.), *Borderline Personality Disorder: Clinical and Empirical Perspectives* (pp. 199–219). New York: Guilford Press.

Ingraham, L. (1995). Family-Genetic research and schizotypal personality. In A. Raine, T. Lencz, and S. Mednick (eds.), *Schizotypal Personality* (pp. 19–42). Cambridge: Cambridge University Press.

Inhelder, B., and Piaget, J. (1958). *The Growth of Logical Thinking.* New York: Basic Books.

Intrator, J., Hare, R. D., Stritske, P., Brichtswein, K., Dorfman, D., Harper, T. J., Bernstein, D., Handelsman, L., Schaefer, C., Keilp, S., Rosen, J., and Machac, S. (1997). A brain imaging (Spect) study of semantic and affective processing in psychopaths. *Biological Psychiatry, 42,* 96–103.

Jacobson, E. (1964). *The self and the object world.* New York: International Universities Press.

Jensen, P., and Hoagwood, K. (1997). The book of names; DSM-IV in context. *Development and Psychopathology 9,* 231–249.

John, O., Caspi, A., Robins, R., Moffitt, T., and Stouthamer-Loeber, M. (1994). The 'little five.' Exploring the nomological network of the five-factor model of personality in adolescent boys. *Child Development, 65,* 160–178.

Kagan, J. (1969). The three faces of continuity in human development. In D. A. Goslin (ed.), *Handbook of Socialization Theory and Research* (pp. 983–1004). Chicago: Rand McNally.

Kagan, J. (1991). The theoretical utility of constructs for self. *Developmental Review, 11,* 244–250.

Kagan, J. (1997). Conceptualizing psychopathology: The importance of developmental profiles. *Development and Psychopathology, 9,* 321–334.

Kagan, J., and H. Moss. (1962). *Birth to Maturity.* New York: John Wiley.

Kagan, J., and Snidman, N. (1991). Tempermental factors in human development. *American Psychologist, 46*(8), 856–862.

Kagan, J., and Zentner, M. (1996). Early childhood predictors of adult psychopathology. *Harvard Review of Psychiatry, 3,* 341–350.

Kahlbaugh, P., and Haviland, J. (1986). Nonverbal communication between parents and adolescents: A study of approach and avoidance behaviors. Special Issue: Development of nonverbal behavior: II. Social development and nonverbal behavior. *Journal of Nonverbal Behavior, 18*(1), 91–113.

Kashani, J., Orvaschel, H., Rosenberg, T., and Reid, J. (1989). Psychopathology: A community sample of children and adolescents: A developmental sample. *Journal of the American Academy of Child and Adolescent Psychiatry, 28,* 701–706.

Keck, J., and Fiebert, M. (1986) Avoidance of anxiety and eating disorders. *Psychological Reports, 58*(2), 432–434.

Kendler, K., McGuire, M., Gruenberg, A., and Walsh, D. (1995). Schizotypal symptoms and signs in the Roscommon Family Study. *Archives of General Psychiatry, 52,* 296–303.

Kernberg, O. (1975). *Borderline Conditions and Pathological Narcissism.* New York: Jason Aronson.

Kernberg, O. (1976). *Object Relations Theory and Clinical Psychoanalysis.* New York: Jason Aronson.

Kernberg, O. (1978). The diagnosis of borderline conditions in adolescence. In S. Feinstein and P. Giovacchini (eds.), *Adolescent Psychiatry, Volume 6, 298–319.* Chicago: University of Chicago Press.

Kernberg, O. (1988/1994). Hysterical and histrionic personality disorders. In R. Michels et al. (eds.), *Psychiatry, 1–11.* Philadelphia: J. B. Lippincott.

Kernberg, O. (1977). The structural diagnosis of borderline personality organization. In *Borderline Personality Disorders: The concept, the syndrome, the patient.* M. P. Hartocollis (ed). New York: I. U. P.

Kernberg, O. (1992). Hysterical and histrionic personality disorders. In *Aggression in Personality Disorders and Perversions* (pp. 52–66). New Haven: Yale University Press.

Kernberg, O. (1996). A psychoanalytic theory of personality disorders. In J. F. Clarkin and M. Lenzenweger (eds.), *Major Theories of Personality Disorder* (pp. 106–137). New York: Guilford Press.

Kernberg, O. F. (1989). The narcissistic personality disorder and the differential diagnosis of antisocial behavior. *Psychiatric Clinics of North America 12(3),* 553–570.

Kernberg, O. F. (1995). Normal and pathological narcissism. In *Borderline Conditions and Pathological Narcissism* (pp. 315–343). New York: Jason Aronson.

Kernberg, P. (1990). Debate forum–Resolved: Borderline personality disorder exists in children under twelve. *Journal of the American Academy of Child and Adolescent Psychiatry, 29,* 478–483.

Kernberg, P. F. (1979). Psychoanalytic profile of the borderline adolescent. *Adolescent Psychiatry, 8,* 234–256.

Kernberg, P. F. (1983). Borderline conditions: Childhood and adolescent aspects, in the borderline child. Robson, K. S., ed. New York: McGraw-Hill, 101–119.

Kernberg, P. F. (1988). Children with borderline personality organization. In C. J. Kestenbaum and D. T. Williams (eds.), *Handbook of Clinical Assessment of Children and Adolescents* (pp. 604–625). New York: New York University Press.

Kernberg, P. F. (1989). Narcissistic personality disorder in childhood. *Psychiatric Clinics of North America, 12(3),* 671–693.

Kernberg, P. F. (1991a). *Children with Conduct Disorders.* New York: Basic Books.

Kernberg, P. F. (1991b). Personality disorders. In J. M. Wiener (ed.), *Textbook of Child and Adolescent Psychiatry* (pp. 515–533). Washington, D.C.: American Psychiatric Press.

Kernberg, P. F. (1994). Mechanisms of defense: Development and research perspectives. *Bulletin of the Menninger Clinic, 58(1),* 55–87.

Kernberg, P. F., Hajal, F., and Normandin, L. (1994). Narcissistic personality disorder in adolescent inpatients–A retrospective record review study of descriptive characteristics. In E. Ronningtram (ed.), *Disorders of Narcissism: Theoretical, Empirical and Clinical Implications* (pp. 437–456). Washington, D.C.: American Psychiatric Press.

Kernberg, P. F., Hajal, F., and Normandin, L. (1998). Narcissistic personality disorders in adolescent inpatients: Descriptive characteristics and treatment issues. In Ronningstam, E. F. (ed.), *Disorders of Narcissism: Theoretical, Empirical, and Clinical Implications*. Washington, D.C.: American Psychiatric Press.

Kernberg, P. F. (1987). Mother-child interaction and mirror behavior. *Infant Mental Health Journal 8*, 4.

Kernberg, P. F., and Chazan, S. L. (1997). *Children's Play Therapy Instrument (CPTI) Manual for Raters*. Unpublished manuscript.

Kernberg, P. F., Chazan, S. L., and Normandin, L. (1998). The Children's Play Therapy Instrument (CPTI). *Journal of Psychotherapy Practice and Research, 7*(3), 196–207.

Kernberg, P. F., Clarkin, A., Greenblatt, E., and Cohen, J. (1992). The Cornell interview of peers and friends: Development of validation. *Journal of American Academy of Child and Adolescent Psychiatry, 31*(3), 483–489.

Kernberg, P. F., and Koenisgberg, H. (1999). *The Extensive Identity Diffusion: On a Particular Form of Identity Diffusion in borderline patients extending the limits of treatability*. A manuscript submitted for publication. New York: Basic Books.

Kestenbaum, C. (1983). Borderline children at risk for major psychiatric disorders in adult life. In K. Robson (ed.), *The Borderline Child* (pp. 49–82). New York: McGraw-Hill.

Knight, R. (1953a). Borderline states. *Bulletin of the Menninger Clinic 17*, 1–12.

Knight, R. P. (1953b). Borderline states. In R. P. Knight and C. R. Friedman (Eds.), *Psychoanalytic psychiatry and psychology*. New York: International Universities Press.

Kohnstamm, G. and Martin, R. (1994). *The Developing Structure of Temperament and Personality from Infancy to Adulthood*. Hillsdale, N.J.: Lawrence Erlbaum.

Kohut, H. (1971). *The Analysis of the Self*. New York: International Universities Press.

Kohut, H. (1972). Thoughts of narcissism and narcissistic Rage. *Psychoanalytic Study of the Child, 27*, 360–400.

Kohut, H. (1980). Diagnosis and treatment of borderline and narcissistic children and adolescents. *Bulletin of the Menninger Clinic, 44*(2), 147–170.

Korner, A. (1967). Significance of primary ego and drive endowment for later development. In J. H. Hellmuth (ed.), *Exceptional Infant, Volume 1: The Normal Infant* (pp. 191–195). New York: Brunner/Mazel.

Krueger, R. F. (1999). Personality traits are linked to crime among men and women: Evidence from a birth cohort. *Journal of Abnormal Psychology, 103*(2), 328–338.

Kruesi, M. (1986). Presentation American Academy of Child Psychiatry.

La Barre, M., and La Barre, W. (1965). The worm in the honeysuckle. *Social Casework, 46*, 399–413.

Laporte, L., and Guttman, H. (1996). Traumatic childhood experiences as risk: Factors for b. l. and other personality disorders. *Journal of Personality Disorders, 10*(3), 247–259.

Last, C. G. (1989). Anxiety disorders of childhood or adolescence. In C. Last and M. Hersen (eds.), *Handbook for Child Psychiatric Diagnosis* (pp. 156–169). New York: John Wiley.

Leichtman, M., and Nathan, S. (1983). A clinical approach to the psychological testing of borderline children. In K. S. Robson (ed.), *The Borderline Child-Approaches to Etiology, Diagnosis, and Treatment* (pp. 121–170). New York: McGraw-Hill.

Leichtman, M., and Shapiro, S. (1980a). An introduction to the psychological assessment of borderline conditions in children: Borderline children and the test process. In J. S. Kwawer et al. (eds.), *Borderline Phenomena and the Rorschach Test* (pp. 353–366). New York: International Universities Press.

Leichtman, M., and Shapiro, S. (1980b). An introduction to the psychological assessment of borderline conditions in children: Manifestations of borderline phenomena on psychological testing. In J. S. Kwawer et al. (Eds.), *Borderline Phenomena and the Rorschach Test* (pp. 367–394). New York: International Universities Press.

Leichtman, M. (1988). When does the Rorschach become the Rorschach? Stages in the mastery of the test. In Lerner, H. and Lerner, P. (Eds.), *Primitive mental states and the Rorschach*. Madison, CT: International Universities Press, 559–600.

Lencz, T., Raine, A., Benishay, D., Mills, S., and Bird, L. (1995). Neuropsychological abnormalities associated with schizotypal personality. In A. Raine, T. Lencz, and S. Mednick (eds.), *Schizotypal Personality* (pp. 289–328). Cambridge: Cambridge University Press.

Lenzenweger, M., Loranger, A. W., Korfine, L. and Neff, C. (1997). Detecting personality disorders in a nonclinical population application of a 2-stage procedure for case identification. *Archives of General Psychiatry, 54*, pp. 345–351.

Lerner, P. (1991). *Psychoanalytic theory and the Rorschach*. Hillsdale, N.J.: The Analytic Press.

Lewinsohn, P., Rohde, P., Seeley, J., and Klein, D. (1997). Axis II psychopathology as a function of Axis I disorders in childhood and adolescence. *Journal of the American Academy of Child and Adolescent Psychiatry, 36*, 1752–1759.

Lewis, M. (1993). The emergence of human emotions. In M. Lewis and J. Haviland (eds.), *Handbook of Emotions* (pp. 223–236). New York: Guilford.

Lewis, M., and Brooks-Gunn, J. (1979). *Social Cognition and the Acquisition of Self*. New York: Plenum Press.

Liebowitz, J. H. (1981). Descriptive aspects and clinical features of borderline children and adolescents: An empirical study. Presented at the American Orthopsychiatric Association, New York City.

Livesley, W. J. (1995). Past achievements and future directions. In W. J. Livesley (ed.), *The DSM-IV Personality Disorders* (pp. 497–506). New York: Guilford.

Livson, N., and Peskin, H. (1967). Prediction of adult psychological health in a longitudinal study. *Journal of Abnormal Psychology, 72*, 509–518.

Llopis Sala, V. R., and Gomez Beneyto, M. (1994). Analysis of factors that influence avoidance behavior in human subjects: An experimental study. *Psiquis, 15*(8), 46–52.

Loeber, R. (1985). The utility of differentiating between mixed and pure forms of antisocial child behavior. *Journal of Abnormal Child Psychology 13*(2): 315–335.

Loranger, A. (1988). *The Personality Disorder Examination (PDE) Manual*. Yonkers, N.Y.: DV Communications.

Loranger, A. W., Oldham, J. M., and Tulis, E. H. (1982). Familial transmission of *DSM-III* borderline personality disorder. *Archives of General Psychiatry, 39*, 795–799.

Loranger, A. W., Sartorius, N., and Andreol, A. (1994). The international personality disorder examination. *Archives of General Psychiatry 51*, 215–223.

Magai, C., and Hunziker, J. (1993). Tolstoy and the riddle of developmental transformation: A lifespan analysis of the role of emotions in personality development. In M. Lewis and J. Haviland (eds.), *Handbook of Emotions* (pp. 247–259). New York: Guilford.

Mahler, M. S. (1971). A study of the separation-individuation process: Its possible application to borderline phenomena in the psychoanalytic situation. *The Psychoanalytic Study of the Child 26*, 403–424.

Mahler, M. S., and Kaplan, L. (1977). Development aspects in the assessment of narcissistic and so-called borderline personalities. In P. Hartcollis (ed.), *Borderline Personality Disorders: The Concept, the Syndrome, the Patient* (pp. 71–85). New York: International Universities Press.

Mahler, M. S., Pine, F., and Bergman, A. (1975) The psychological birth of the human infant. New York: Basic Books.

Mahler, M. S., Ross, J. R., Jr., and DeFries, Z. (1949). Clinical studies in benign and malignant cases of childhood psychosis (schizophrenia-like). *American Journal of Orthopsychiatry, 19*, 295–305.

Main, M. (1993). Discourse, prediction and recent studies in attachment: Implications for psychoanalysis. *Journal of the American Psychoanalytic Association, 41* (5), 209–244.

Main, M., and R. Goldwyn. (1994). *Adult Attachment Scoring and Classification Systems.* London: University College.

March, J. S., and Mulle, K. (1998). *OCD in Children and Adolescents: A Cognitive-Behavior Treatment Manual.* New York: Guilford.

Marcia, J. E. (1966). Development and validation of ego identity status. *Journal of Personality and Social Psychology, 3*, 351–358.

Mariategui, J. (1970). Estudios de epidemiologia psiquiatrica en el Peru. In J. Mariategui and G. Adis Castro (Eds.), *Epidemiologia Psiquiatrica en America Latina.* Buenos Aires: Acta Fondo para la Salud Mental.

Martin, R., Wisenbaker, J., and Huttunen, M. (1994). Review of factor analytic studies of temperament measures based on the Thomas-Chess structural model: Implications for the Big Five. In C. Halverson Jr., G. Kohnstamm, and R. Martin (eds.), *The Developing Structure of Temperament and Personality from Infancy to Adulthood* (pp. 157–172). Hillsdale, N.J.: Lawrence Erlbaum.

Matheny, A. (1989). Children's behavioral inhibition over age and across situations: Genetic similarity for a trait during a change. Special Issue: Long-term stability and change in personality. *Journal of Personality, 57*(2), 215–235.

McCall, R. (1979). The development of intellectual functioning in infancy and the prediction of later IQ. In J. Osofsky (ed.), *Handbook of Infant Development*, 707–741. New York: John Wiley.

McGlashan, T. (1986). Schizotypal personality disorder: Chestnut Lodge follow-up study. VI: Long term follow-up perspectives. *Archives of General Psychiatry, 43,* 329–334.

McGlashan, T. H. (1983). The borderline syndrome II. Is it a variant of schizophrenia or affective disorder? *Archives of General Psychiatry, 40,* 319–323.

Mednick, S., Parnas, J., and Schulsinger, F. (1987). The Copenhagen High-Risk Project, 1962–1986. *Schizophrenia Bulletin, 13,* 485–495.

Mednick, S. A., Gabrielli, W. F., and Hutchings, B. (1984). Genetic influences in criminal behavior: Some evidence from an adoption cohort. *Science, 224,* 891–893.

Meehl, P. E. (1990). Towards an integrated theory of schizotaxia, schizotypy, and schizophrenia. *Journal of Personaltiy Disorders, 4,* 1–99.

Mehlum, L., Friis, S., Irion, T., Johns, S., Karterud, S., Vaglum, P., and Vaglum, S. (1991). Personality disorders 2–5 years after treatment: A prospective follow-up study. *Acta Psychiatrica Scandanavia, 84,* 72–77.

Meloy, J. R., and Gacono, C. B. (1998). The internal world of the psychopath. In T. Millon, E. Simonsen, and D. Birket Smith (eds.), *Psychopathy, Antisocial, Criminal and Violent Behavior* (pp. 95–109). New York: Guilford Press.

Meltzer, Donald (1975). Adhesive identification. *Contemporary Psychoanalysis 11*(3), 289–310.

Merikangas, K., and Weissman, M. (1986). Epidemiology of *DSM-III* Axis II personality disorders. In A. Frances and R. Hales (eds.), *APA Annual Review (Vol. 5)* (pp. 258–278). Washington, D.C.: American Psychiatric Press.

Metcalf, A. (1977). Childhood process to structure. In M. J. Horowitz (ed.), *Hysterical Personality.* New York: Jason Aronson.

Metcalf, A. (1991). Childhood process to structure. In M. J. Horowitz (ed.), *Hysterical Personality Style and the Histrionic Personality Disorder,* rev. ed. (pp. 69–145). New York: Jason Aronson.

Millon, T. (1969). Modern Psychopathology: A biosocial approach to maladaptive learning and functioning. Philadelphia: Saunders.

Million, T., and Davis, R. (1995). The development of personality disorders. In D. Cicchetti and D. Cohen (Eds.), *Developmental Psychopathology.* New York: J. Wiley and Sons, 633–676.

Moffitt, T., Caspi, A., Dickson, N., Silva, P., and Stanton, W. (1996). Childhood-Onset versus adolescent-onset antisocial conduct problems in males: Natural history from ages 3 to 18 years. *Development and Psychopathology, 8,* 399–425.

Moffitt, T. E. (1993). Adolescence-Limited and life course–persistent antisocial behavior: A developmental view. *Psychological Review, 100*(46), 674–701.

Morey, L. C. (1988). Personality disorders under *DSM-III* and *DSM-III-R*: An examination of convergence, coverage and internal consistency. *American Journal of Psychiatry, 145,* 573–577.

Moss, E., Parent, S., and Gosselin, C. (1995). Attachment and theory of mind: Cognitive and metacognitive correlates of attachment during the preschool period. Paper presented at the biennial meeting of the Society for Research in Child Development.

Myers, W. (1995). Psychopathology, biopsychosocial factors, crime characteristics, and classification of twenty-five homicidal youths. *Journal of the American Academy of Child and Adolescent Psychiatry 34* (11), 1483–1489.

Nagera, H. (1969). The imaginary companion: Its significance for ego development and conflict solution. *The Psychoanalytic Study of the Child, 24,* 165–175.

National Advisory Mental Health Council. (1995). *Basic Behavioral Science Research for Mental Health.* Washington, D.C.: U.S. Department of Health and Human Services, National Institutes of Health Publication No. 95–3682.

Naziroglu, F., McKay, D., Todoro, J., and Yaryura-Tobias, J. (1996). Effect of cognitive behavior therapy on persons with body dysmorphic disorder and comorbid Axis II diagnosis. *Behavior Therapy, 27*(1), 67–77.

Noshpitz, J. (1993). Verbal communication.

Olin, S., Raine, A., Cannon, T., Parnas, J., Schulsinger, F., and Mednick, S. (1997). Childhood behavior precursors of schizotypal personality disorder. *Schizophrenia Bulletin, 23,* 93–103.

Pajer, K.A. (1998). What happens to "bad" girls: A review of the adult outcome of antisocial adolescent girls. *American Journal of Psychiatry, 155*(7), 862–870.

Paris, J. (1994). Borderline personality disorder: a multidimensional approach. Washington, DC: American Psychiatric Press.

Paris, J. (1996). *Social Factors in the Personality Disorders.* Cambridge: Cambridge University Press.

Parker, Z., and Stewart, E. (1994). School consultation and the management of obsessive-compulsive personality in the classroom. *Adolescence, 29*(115), 563–574.

Patrick, M., Hobson, R. P., Castle, D., Howard, R., and Maughan, B. (1994). Personality disorder and the mental representation of early social experience. *Development and Psychopathology, 6,* 375–388.

Pennington, B., and Ozonoff, S. (1996) Executive functions and developmental psychopathology. *Journal of Child Psychology and Psychiatry, 37*(1), 51–87.

Perry, C., Kardos, M., and Pagano, C. (1993). The study of defenses in psychotherapy using the Defense Mechanism Rating Scale (DMRS). In U. Hentschel and W. Ehlers (eds.), *The Concept of Defense Mechanisms in Comtemporary Psychology: Theoretical, Research, and Clinical Perspectives* (pp. 122–132). New York: Springer.

Perry, J. C. (1990). Psychological defense mechanisms and the study of affective and anxiety disorder. In S. D. Maser and C. R. Cloninger (eds.), *Comorbidity of Mood and Anxiety Disorders* (pp. 545–562). Washington, D.C.: American Psychiatric Press.

Perry, J. C. (1993). Longitudinal studies of personality disorders. *Journal of Personality Disorders, Supplement,* 68–85.

Perry, J. C., Hoglend, P., Shear, K., Vaillant, G., Horowitz, M., Kardos, M. E., Bille-Henrik, M. D., and Kazan, D. (1998). Field trial of a diagnostic axis for defense mechanisms for *DSM-IV. Journal of Personality Disorders, 12*(1), 156–168.

Petti, T. A. (1981). Borderline psychotic behavior in hospitalized children: Approaches to assessment and treatment. *Journal of the American Academmy of Child Psychiatry, 21*, 197–202.

Pfeffer, C. R. (1982). Clinical observations of suicidal behavior in a neurotic, a borderline, and a psychotic child: Common processes of symptom formation. *Child Psychiatry and Human Development, 13*(2), 120–134.

Piaget, J. (1950). *The Psychology of Intelligence.* New York: Harcourt, Brace.

Pine, F. (1983). A working nosology of borderline syndromes in children. In K. S. Robson (Ed.), *The borderline child—Approaches to etiology, diagnosis, and treatment.* New York: McGraw-Hill, 83–100.

Pine, F. (1974). On the concept 'borderline' in children: A clinical essay. *Psychoanalyitic Study Child 29*: 391–398.

Plutchik, R. (1993). Emotions and their vicissitudes: Emotions and psychopathology. In M. Lewis and J. Haviland (eds.), *Handbook of Emotions* (pp. 53–66). New York: Guilford.

Pope, H. G., et al. (1983). The validity of *DSM-III* borderline personality disorder. *Archives of General Psychiatry, 40*, 23–29.

Post, R. M., Rubinow, D. R., Ballenger, J. C. (1984). Conditioning, sensitization, and kindling: Implications for the course of affective illness, in neurobiology of mood disorders. Baltimore, M.D.: Williams & Wilkins, 432–466.

Price, B. H., Daffner, K. R., Stowe, R. M., and Mesulam, M. M. (1990). The compartmental learning disabilities of early frontal lobe damage. *Brain, 113*, 1383–1393.

Raine, A., Lencz, T., and Mednick, S. (Eds.), (1995). *Schizotypal personality.* Cambridge, England: University of Cambridge Press.

Rappaport, D., Gill, M., and Schafer, R. (1968). Diagnostic psychological testing. New York: International Universities Press.

Reister, G., and Schepank, H. (1989). Anxiety and depression in an urban population: Results of the Mannheim Cohort study. *Psychiatric Psychobiology 4*, 299–306.

Rie, H. (1966). Depression in childhood. *Journal of the American Academy of Child Psychiatry 5*, 653–686.

Rinsley, D. (1989). Notes on the developmental pathogenesis of narcissistic personality disorder. *The Psychiatric Clinics of North America, 12*, 695–707.

Rinsley, D. B. (1980a). The development etiology of borderline and narcissistic disorders. *Bulletin of the Menninger Clinic, 44*, 127–134.

Rinsley, D. B. (1980b). Diagnosis and treatment of borderline and narcissistic children and adolescents. *Bulletin of the Menninger Clinic, 44*, 147–170.

Rinsley, D. B. (1981). Borderline psychopathology: The concepts of Masterson and Rinsley and beyond. *Adolescent Psychiatry I, 9*, 259–274.

Robbins, L. (1966). Childhood behavior predicting later diagnosis. In *Deviant Children Grown Up: A Sociological and Psychiatric Study of Sociopathic Personality* (pp. 135–158). Baltimore: Williams and Wilkins.

Robins and Regier (1991). Cross-cultural feasibility, reliability and sources of variance of the Composite International Diagnostic Interview (CIDI). *British Journal of Psychiatry 159*, 645–653.

Robson, K. S. (1983). *The Borderline Child—Approaches to Etiology, Diagnosis, and Treatment.* New York: McGraw-Hill.

Rodriguez Torres, A., and Del Porto, J. A. (1995). Comorbidity of obsessive-compulsive disorder and personality disorders: A Brazilian controlled study. *Psychopathology, 28*(6), 322–329.

Ronningstam, E. F. (1998). Narcissistic personality disorder and pathological narcissism. In Ronningstam, E. F. (ed.), *Disorders of Narcissism: Theoretical, Empirical, and Clinical Implications* (pp. 375–413). Washington, D.C.: American Psychiatric Press.

Roseby, V., Erdberg, R., Bardenstein, K., and Johnston, K. (1995). Developmental psychopathology in children in high-conflict families: Attachment, personality disorders and the Rorschach. Paper presented at the Convention of the Society for Research in Child Development, Kansas City.

Rosenfeld, K., and Sprince, M. (1963). An attempt to formulate the meaning of the concept "borderline." *The Psychoanalytic Study of the Child*, 603–635.

Rothbart, M., Ahadi, S., and Hershey, K. (1994). Temperament and social behavior in childhood. *Merrill-Palmer Quarterly, 40*, 21–39.

Rothbart, M., Posner, M., and Hershey, K. (1995). Temperament, attention, and developmental psychopathology. In D. Cicchetti and D. Cohen (eds.), *Developmental Psychopathology* (pp. 315–342). New York: John Wiley.

Rourke, B. (1989). *Syndrome of Nonverbal Learning Disability.* New York: Guilford.

Rourke, B., Fisk, J., and Strang, J. (1986). *Neuropsychological Assessment of Children.* New York: Guilford.

Ruegg, R., and Frances, A. (1995). New research in personality disorders. *Journal of Personality Disorders, 9*, 1–48.

Rutter, M. (1987). Temperament, personality, and personality disorder. *British Journal of Psychiatry, 150*, 443–458.

Rygaard, N. P. (1998). Psychopathic children: Indicators of organic dysfunction in psychopathy. In T. Millon, E. Simonsen, M. Burket-Smith, and R. D. Davis (eds.), *Psychopathy: Antisocial, criminal, and violent behavior*, 247–259. New York: Guilford.

Sadock, J. H., Kaplan, T., and Freedman, M. (1976). *The Sexual Experience.* Baltimore: Williams and Wilkins.

Sandler, J. (1976). Countertransference and role responsiveness. *International Journal of Psychoanalysis, 3*, 43–48.

Sandler, J., and Rosenblatt, B. (1962). The concept of the representational world. *Psychoanalytic Study of the Child 17*: 128–145. New Haven: Yale University Press.

Schaefer, C. E., and Millman, H. L. (1994). *How to Help Children with Common Problems.* New York: Jason Aronson.

Schubert, D. L., Sacuzzo, D. P., and Braff, B. L. (1985). Information in borderline patients. *Journal of Nervous and Mental Disorders 173* (1): 26–31.

Schwartz, L., and Eagle, C. (1986). *Psychological Portraits of Children.* Lexington, MA: D.C. Heath & Co.

Seligman, M. E. (1975). *Helpless*. San Francisco: W. J. Freeman.

Selman, R. (1980). *The Growth of Interpersonal Understanding, Development and Clinical Analyses*. New York: Academic Press.

Selzer, M. A., Kernberg, P. F., Fibel, B., Cherbuliez, T., Mortati, S. (1987). The personality assessment interview: preliminary review. *Psychiatry, 50*(2), 142–153.

Senn, M. J. E., and Solnit, A. J. (1968). *Problems in child behavior and development*. Philadelphia: Lea and Febiger.

Settlage, C. F. (1977). The psychoanalytic understanding of narcissistic and borderline personalities: Advances in developmental theory. *Journal of the American Psychoanalytic Association, 25*, 805–833.

Shapiro, E. R., Zinner, J., Shapiro, R. L., and Berkowitz, D. A. (1975). The influence of family experience on borderline personality development. *Int. Rev. Psychoanal. 2*: 399–412.

Shapiro, T. (1990). Debate orum–Resolved: Borderline personality disorder exists in children under twelve. *Journal of the American Academy of Child and Adolescent Psychiatry, 29*, 478–483.

Sherwood, V. (1994). Psychotherapy of the quiet borderline patient: the as-if personality revisited, 289–294. Northbale, N.J.: J. Aronson.

Siever, L. S., and Davie, K. L. (1991). A psychobiological perspective on the personality disorders. *American Journal of Psychiatry, 148*, 1647–1658.

Slater, A. (1995). Individual differences in infancy and later IQ. *Journal of Child Psychology and Psychiatry, 36*, 69–112.

Sloate, P. (1998). The role of auditory defenses in the treatment of a narcissistic boy. In P. E. Beren (ed.), *Narcissistic Disorders in Children and Adolescents: Diagnoses and Treatment* (pp. 187–212). New York: Jason Aronson.

Smith, A. H., Gacono, C. B., and Kaufman, L. (1997). A Rorschach comparison of psychopathic and non-psychopathic conduct disordered adolescents. *Journal of Clinical Psychology, 53*(4), 289–300.

Soldz, S., Budman, S., Demby, A., and Merry, J. (1995). The relation of defensive style to personality pathology and the big five personality factors. *Journal of Personality Disorders, 9*(4), 356–370.

Soloff, H. P., and Millward, J. W. (1983). Developmental histories of borderline patients. *Comprehensive Psychiatry 24*(6): 574–588.

Sperling, M. (1973). Conversion hysteria and conversion symptoms. *American Psychoanalytic Association, 21*, 745–771.

Squires-Wheeler, E., Friedman, D., Amminger, G. P., Skodol, A., Looser-Ott, S., Roberts, S., Pape, S., and Erlinmeyer-Kimling, S. (1997). Negative and positive dimensions of schizotypal personality disorder. *Journal of Personality Disorders, 11*, 285–300.

Squires-Wheeler, E., Skodol, A., and Erlenmeyer-Kimling, L. (1992). The assessment of of schizotypal features over two points in time. *Schizophrenia Research, 6*, 75–85.

Squires-Wheeler, E., Skodol, A., Friedman, D., and Erlenmeyer-Kimling, L. (1989). *DSM-III-R* schizotypal personality traits in offspring of schziophrenic disorder, affective disorder, and normal control parents. *Journal of Psychiatric Reserach, 23*, 229–239.

Sroufe, A. (1997). Psychopathology as an outcome of development. *Development and Psychopathology,* 9, 251–268.

Sroufe, A., Carlson, E., and Schulman, S. (1993). Individuals in relationships: Development from infancy through adolescence. In D. Funder, R. Parke, C. Tomilson-Keasey, and K. Widaman (Eds.), *Studying Lives Through Time* (pp. 315–342). Washington, D.C.: American Psychological Association.

Steiner, H., and Feldman, S. (1997). Two Approaches to the Measurement of Adaptive Style: Comparison of Normal Psychosomatically Ill and Delinquent Adolescence. Unpublished manuscript.

Stern, D. F. (1985). *The Interpersonal World of the Infant: A view from psychoanalysis and developmental psychology.* New York: Basic Books.

Stone, M. (1993a). *Abnormalities of Personality: Within and Beyond the Realm of Treatment.* New York: W. W. Norton.

Stone, M. (1998). Sadistic personality in murderers. In T. Millon, E. Simonsen, and D. Birket-Smith (Eds.), *Psychopathy* (pp. 347–355). New York: Guilford.

Stone, M. H. (1993b). Long term outcome in personality disorders. *British Journal of Psychiatry,* 162, 299–313.

Stone, M. H. (1990). *The Fate of Borderline Patients: Successful Outcome and Psychiatric Practice.* New York: Guilford.

Strauss, C. (1990). Overanxious disorder in childhood. In M. Hersen and C. G. Last (eds.), *Handbook of Child and Adult Psychopathology: A Longitudinal Perspective* (pp. 237–246). New York: Pergamon Press.

Teicher, M. H., Ito, Y., Glod, C. A., Schiffer, F., and Gelbard, H. (1994). Early childhood abuse and limbic system ratings in adult psychiatric outpatients. *Journal of Neuropsychiatry and Clinical Neurosciences* 5 (3): 301–306.

Thomas, A., and Chess, S. (1977). *Temperament and Development.* New York: Brunner/Mazel.

Thompson, M., Asarnow, J., Hamilton, E. B., Newell, L., Turner, S., Beidel, D., Dancu, C. V., and Keys, K. J. (1986). Psychopathology of social phobia and comparison to avoidant personality disorder. *Journal of Abnormal Psychology,* 95, 389–394.

Turner, S., Beidel, D., Bordon, J. W., Stanley, M. R., and Jacob, R. G. (1991). Social phobia: Axis I and Axis II correlates. *Journal of Abnormal Psychology,* 100, 102–106.

Tyrer, P. (1995). Are personality disorders well classified in DSM-IV? In W. J. Livesley (Ed.), *The DSM-IV Personality Disorders.* New York: Guilford.

Tyrer, P., Casey, P., and Ferguson, B. (1991). Personality disorders in perspective. *British Journal of Psychiatry,* 159, 463–471.

Vaillant, G. E. (1979). *Adaptation to life.* Boston: Little, Brown.

Vaillant, G. E., Bond, M., and Vaillant, C. O. (1986). An empirically validated hierarchy of defense mechanisms. *Archives of General Psychiatry,* 43, 786–794.

Van der Kolk, B. A., and Greenberg, M. S. (1987). The psychobiology of the trauma response: Hyperarousal, constrition, and addiction to traumatic reexposure, in Psychological Trauma. Washington, D.C.: American Psychiatric Press, 63–87.

Vela, R., Gottlieb, E., and Gottlieb, H. (1983). Borderline syndromes in childhood: A critical review. In K. S. Robson (Ed.). *The Borderline Child—Approaches to etiology, Diagnosis, and Treatment,* 31–48. New York: McGraw-Hill.

Verhulst, F. C. (1984). Diagnosing borderline children. *Acta Paedopsychiat 50:* 161–173.

Volkvan, V. D. (1979). The glass bubble of the narcissistic patient in advances. In Capponi, L. J. (Ed.), *Psychotherapy of the Borderline patient.* New York: Jason Aronson.

Wachs, T. (1994). Fit, context, and the transition between temperament and personality. In C. Halverson Jr., G. Kohnstamm, and R. Martin (eds.), *The Developing Structure of Temperament and Personality from Infancy to Adulthood* (pp. 209–220). Hillsdale, N.J.: Lawrence Erlbaum.

Walker, E., and Gale, S. (1995). Neurodevelopmental processes in schizophrenia and schizotypal personality disorder. In A. Raine, T. Lencz, and S. Mednick (eds.), *Schizotypal Personality* (pp. 56–75). Cambridge: Cambridge University Press.

Wallerstein, R. S. (1983). Defenses, defense mechanisms and the structure of the mind. *Journal of the American Psychoanalytic Association, 31* (Supplement), 201–225.

Wallerstein, R. S. (1998). Erikson's concept of ego identity reconsidered. *Journal of the American Psychoanalytic Association, 46*(1), 229–247.

Weil, A. P. (1953). Certain severe disturbances of ego development in childhood. *The Psychoanalytic Study of the Child 8,* 271–287.

Weiner, I. (1986a). Assessing children and adolescents with the Rorschach. In H. Knoff (Ed.), *The Assessment of Child and Adolescent Personality* (pp. 141–172). New York: Guilford.

Weiner, I. B. (1986b). Conceptual and empirical perspectives on the Rorschach assessment of psychopathology. *Journal of Personality Assessment 50,* 472–479.

Weintraub, S., and Mesulam, M. (1983). Developmental learning disabilities of the right hemisphere: Emotional, interpersonal, and cognitive components. *Archives of Neurology, 40,* 463–468.

Weiss, M., Zelkowitz, P., Vogel, S., Guzder, S., Heyman, M., Feldman, R., and Paris, J. (1995). Children of mothers with borderline personality disorder. *Comprehensive Psychiatry 36*(2): 157–163.

Weissman, M. (1993). The epidemiology of personality disorders: A 1990 update. *Journal of Personality Disorders, Supplement,* 44–62.

Wells, K. C., and Forehand, R. (1985). Conduct and oppositional disorders. In P. H. Bornstein and A. E. Kazdin (eds.), *Handbook of Clinical Behavior Therapy with Children* (pp. 218–265). Homewood, IL: Dorsey.

White, J. (1990). The neuropsychology of delinquency: A critical review of theory and research. In N. Morris and M. Tonty (eds.), *Crime and Justice, Volume 12* (pp. 99–169). Chicago: University of Chicago Press.

White, J., and Silva, P. A. (1988). IQ and delinquency: A direct test of the differential detection hypothesis. *Journal of the American Academy of Child and Adolescent Psychiatry, 27,* 233–240.

White, J., Moffitt, T. E., Earls, F. Robins, L. N., and Silva, D. A. (1990). How early can we tell? Preschool predictors of boys' conduct disorder and delinquency. *Criminology, 28,* 507–533.

Widiger, T., and Trull, T. (1992). Personality and psychopathology: An application of the Five-Factor Model. *Journal of Personality, 60,* 365–393.

Widiger, T., Frances, A., Warner, L., and Bluhm, C. (1986). Diagnostic criteria for the borderline and schizotypal personality disorders. *Journal of Abnormal Psychology,* *95*, 43–51.

Widiger, T. A., and Allen, F. J. (1988). Personality disorders. In J. A. Talbott, R. E. Hales, and S. C. Yudofsky (eds.), *Textbook of Psychiatry* (pp. 631–632). Washington, D.C.: American Psychiatric Press.

Wolff, S. (1991). "Schizoid" personality in childhood and adult life—I: The vagaries of diagnostic labelling. *British Journal of Psychiatry, 159,* 615–620.

Wolff, P. H. (1959). Observations on new born infants. *Psychosomatic Medicine, 21,* 110–118.

Wolff, S. (1991) "Schizoid" personality in childhood and adult life–III: The childhood picture. *British Journal of Psychiatry, 159,* 629–635.

Wolff, S., Townshend, R., McGuire, R., and Weeks, D. (1991). "Schizoid" personality in childhood and adult life–II: Adult adjustment and the continuity with schizotypal personality disorder. *British Journal of Psychiatry, 159,* 620–629.

World Health Organization. (1995). *International Personality Disorder Examination (IPDE) DSM-IV Module.* Washington, D.C.: American Psychiatric Press.

Zanarini, M. C., Gunderson, J. G., and Marino, M. F. (1989). Childhood experiences of borderline patients. *Comprehensive Psychiatry, 30,* 18–25.

Zetzel, E. (1968). The so-called good hysteric. *Int. J. Psychoanal., 49,* 256–260.

Index

Continuity, 40. *See also* Stability
Contracting, 217–218
Conversion, 101
Coping Deficit Index (CDI), 78, 117, 187
Coping, 56, 149–150
Costa, Paul, 18, 248
Countertransference, 192, 212–213
Covert antisocial behavior, 202
CPTI. *See* Children's Play Therapy Instrument
Criminals. *See* Offenders (criminal)
Cultural practices, 105–106
Culture and personality disorders, 247–248

Dahl, A. A., 156
Danish High-Risk Study, 231
Daydreams, 213–214
Deafness, 185
De-animation, 65
Deceitfulness, 194
Dedifferentiation, 64–65
Defense mechanisms, 16, 28–29, 56–68, 104–105, 107, 123, 255–257
  borderline personality disorder, 149–150, 165–166
  narcissistic personality disorder, 191
  psychotic, 165–166, 226
Defensive behaviors, 28–29
D'Elia, F., 111
Delinquent Behavior Index, 94
Denial, 62
Dependent personality disorder, 38
DEPI. *See* Depression Index
Depression Index (DEPI), 187
Derryberry, D., 19–21, 26
Development
  aberrant, 164
  arrested, 164
  emotional, 77
  and personality disorders, 7–14, 35–38
Developmental analysis, 75–76
Developmental psychopathology
  antisocial personality disorder, 206–207
  avoidant personality disorder, 115–116

borderline personality disorder, 141–147
hysterical personality disorder, 102–108
narcissistic personality disorder, 182–187
obsessive-compulsive personality disorder, 122–123
Deviant verbalizations, 73
Diaferia, G., 120–121
Diagnosis
  and antisocial personality disorder, 200–206, 211
  and avoidant personality disorder, 120
  and hysterical personality disorder, 112–114
  and narcissistic personality disorder, 187–188
  of personality disorders, 6–7, 253–254
Diagnostic and Statistical Manual of Mental Disorders (DSM), 4, 5–6, 13–14, 33, 36, 251–253. *See also* Axis I disorders; Axis II disorders
Diagnostic Interview Schedule for Children (DISC), 55–56
Differential diagnosis. *See* Diagnosis
Digman, J., 18–19
DISC. *See* Diagnostic Interview Schedule for Children
Dismantling, 65–66
Disordered thinking, 8
Dispersal, 65
Disregard for safety, 196
Distinctness of state, 103
Divorce, 249–251
Dog phobias, 111
Doing and undoing, 60
Dramatic-emotional cluster, 34
Draw-a-Person, 150
Drawings, 80
Dreams, 213–214
Drug intervention. *See* Pharmacological intervention

Easser, B. R., 99
Ebata, A., 111
Eccentric cluster, 34, 227

Mesulam, M., 243
Metcalf, A., 105–106
Millman, H. L., 115, 121
Millward, J. W., 156, 157, 159
Minnesota Multiphasic Personality
   Inventory (MMPI), 154–155
Mirroring, 167
MMPI. *See* Minnesota Multiphasic
   Personality Inventory
Mode reliance, 103
Moffitt, T. E., 201, 203, 204, 205, 252–253
Moos, R., 111
Mother-child attachment bond, 105, 160.
   See also Parents
Motivational Systems, 19–20
Mulle, K., 124
Murder, 193, 198
Mutism, 11–12, 114

Name identification, 7
Narcissism, 14, 180–182
Narcissistic personality disorder
   (NPD), 37, 93–99, 131–132,
   179–192
Negation, 60
NEO-PI-R. *See* Revised NEO Personality
   Inventory
Neurobiological model, 156
Neurological development, 155
Neuropsychological developmental
   disorders, 15, 26–28
Neuropsychological Screening Tasks,
   150
Neurotic domain, 56, 138–139
Neuroticism, 18
Neurotic personality organization,
   49–51, 83–84
New York Longitudinal Study, 17–18
New Zealand Longitudinal Study,
   205
"Nonorganic" borderlines, 156
Nonverbal learning disability
   syndrome, 27
Normal domain, 56
Normandin, L., 256
Noshpitz, J., 210
NPD. *See* Narcissistic personality
   disorder

Object Relations Theory, 22
Object-representation, 50, 52, 54–55, 78,
   154, 160–161
Obsessive-compulsive disorder (OCD),
   120–121
Obsessive-compulsive personality
   disorder (OCPD), 83–84, 119–128
OCD. *See* Obsessive-compulsive
   disorder
OCPD. *See* Obsessive-compulsive
   personality disorder
Odd-eccentric cluster, 34, 227
Oedipal situations, 163–164, 172
Offenders (criminal), 203–204
Omnipotent control, 64
Openness, 18
Operational reasoning system, 8
Oppositional Disorder, 252
"Organic" borderlines, 156
Organization of temperament, 17–18
Overt antisocial behavior, 202

PAI. *See* Personality Assessment
   Interview
Paranoid personalities, 142
Paranoid personality disorder (PPD), 38,
   227–229, 236–238
Parents
   and avoidant disorder, 115–116
   and borderline personality disorder,
      171–172
   and OCPD, 122–123
   See also Divorce; Families; Mother-
      child attachment bond
Parker, Z., 121, 124
Patrick, M., 25
Patterns of interaction, 10–11
PDE. *See* Personality Disorder
   Examination
PDs. *See* Personality disorders
Peak excitement, 103–104
Peer relationships. *See* Friendship
Perry, J. C., 14, 28, 256
Personality, 6
   components of, 15–32
   development of, 257–258
   emergence of, 7–8
   and stability, 8–11